# Hospital-acquired Infection
**Principles and Prevention**

Second edition

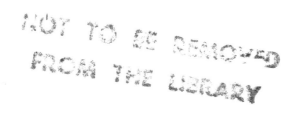

# Hospital-acquired Infection
## Principles and Prevention

Second edition

**G A J Ayliffe**   MD, FRCPath
Professor of Medical Microbiology, Birmingham University; Honorary Director, Hospital
Infection Research Laboratory, Dudley Road Hospital, Birmingham

**B J Collins**
Late Chief Medical Laboratory Scientific Officer, Hospital Infection Research Laboratory,
Dudley Road Hospital, Birmingham

**L J Taylor**
Division of Hospital Infection, Central Public Health Laboratory Service, London

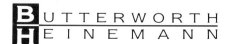

Butterworth–Heinemann Ltd
Westbury House, Bury Street, Guildford, Surrey GU2 5BH

 PART OF REED INTERNATIONAL BOOKS

OXFORD   LONDON   GUILDFORD   BOSTON
MUNICH   NEW DELHI   SINGAPORE   SYDNEY
TOKYO   TORONTO   WELLINGTON

First published by John Wright and Sons Ltd 1982
Reprinted 1983
Second edition 1990
Reprinted 1991

**British Library Cataloguing in Publication Data**
Ayliffe, G. A. J.
  Hospital-acquired infection. 2nd ed.
  1. Hospital. Patients. Nosocomial infections, control
  I. Title II. Collins, B. J.   III. Taylor, Lynda
  614.4′4

ISBN 0 7506 1560 5

**Library of Congress Cataloguing in Publication Data**
Ayliffe, G. A. J.
  Hospital-acquired infection: principles and prevention/
  G. A. J. Ayliffe, B. J. Collins, L. J. Taylor. – 2nd ed.
    p.   cm.
  Includes bibliographical references.
  ISBN 0–7506–1560–5
  1. Nosocomial infections – Prevention.   2. Hospitals
  – Disinfection.   3. Hospitals – Sanitation.
  I. Collins, B. J.   II. Taylor, L. J.
  III. Title
  RA969.A95   1990
  614.4′8–dc20

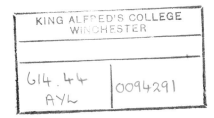
Printed in Great Britain by Cambridge University Press

# Foreword

Textbooks must be kept up-to-date by periodic revision to incorporate new knowledge and new techniques; an extra reason for revising a book on the control of infection is to report biological changes, including new patterns and mechanisms of antibiotic resistance, newly discovered modes of transmission, and even new diseases. Many of these changes reflect the emergence, by selection, of microbial variants better able to resist our efforts in hospital to keep virulent pathogens away from susceptible patients; they will, in varying measure, offset the benefits of improved treatment and prophylaxis; the arrival of a new disease will, in addition, cause widespread alarm and uncertainty. Just when the medical world was congratulating itself on a great triumph, the eradication of smallpox, it suffered a blow that was, perhaps, even greater – the appearance and pandemic spread of the human immunodeficiency virus (HIV) and of AIDS for which there was, and still is, neither cure nor vaccine. It was a disaster that sadly offset the triumphs recently scored against many other types of infection.

These newly arrived community infections were not featured in the first edition of this book. In this new edition Professor Ayliffe and his co-authors consider the possible threat which they pose to staff and patients in hospital. Their comments, the facts they present, and the advice they give should allay some of the worst anxieties of staff exposed to possible contamination by the HIV; as they point out, this blood-borne virus is less easily transmitted and more sensitive to disinfectants than the hepatitis B virus, for the control of which valuable guidelines have been available for some time.

The basic principles and practice of hospital infection control have not been altered by the dramatic incursion of the HIV. This edition again emphasizes the use of methods established by scientific assessment and the avoidance of traditional but ineffective 'rituals'. The contents are similar to those of the first edition, up-dated in various respects, with some improvements in layout and the insertion of newly developed procedures, e.g. topical treatment with mupirocin for nasal carriers of methicillin-resistant *Staphylococcus aureus,* improved methods of cleaning and disinfection of endoscopes, and advice on the use of pre-cooked chilled food in hospitals. The recommendations are compact and clearly presented, reflecting the authors' long personal involvement in the practice of infection control and of studies at the Hospital Infection Research Laboratory. This edition, like its forerunner, will be of the greatest value to a wide spectrum of hospital workers.

**E. J. L. Lowbury** DM, FRCPath

# Preface to the second edition

New problems in hospital infection have arisen since the publication of the first edition. Methicillin-resistant *Staphylococcus aureus* have been causing increasing infections all over the world. The prevention of the spread of these organisms has increased the need for effective isolation procedures and the provision of suitable isolation facilities in individual hospitals. Outbreaks of legionnaires' disease have occurred, and have often been due to inadequate maintenance of cooling towers and water supply systems. However, the predominant anxiety has been the emergence of the human immunodeficiency virus (HIV). Although there have been few reports of transmission to health care staff, the risk, however remote, of developing AIDS has led to a reconsideration of methods of avoiding blood-borne infection. The precautions introduced have often been unnecessarily extreme, and not based on the actual risk, which is low in most hospitals. The potential risk has involved new studies on methods of decontamination of equipment and surfaces. For similar reasons, the overall hazards of infection to hospital staff have received increasing attention, as have the risks of food poisoning to staff and patients, particularly in relation to cook–chill systems.

Nevertheless, these recent problems still represent a small part of the overall problem of hospital infection; of the 10% of infections acquired by patients, most are still of surgical wounds, urinary or the respiratory tract. The cost of infection has to be considered carefully by Infection Control Staff. New control measures have to be cost-effective. This should involve the detection of high risk patients and concentrating resources on these rather than spreading the rather limited resources equally over the whole hospital.

The basic principles of infection control have changed very little and all hospital staff need to be taught these principles, and a major task of Infection Control Doctors and Nurses is to produce, implement and monitor effective policies.

It is hoped that this new edition will continue to provide staff with an understanding of hospital-acquired infection. Although the book is primarily an introduction for Infection Control Nurses and microbiologists, much of the information should be useful to other grades of staff as indicated in the preface to the first edition.

**G. A. J. Ayliffe**

# Preface to the first edition

Although a number of excellent books on the control of hospital infection are now available, few provide evidence or discuss reasons for making decisions. The Hospital Infection Research Laboratory (Regional Health Service Infection Research Laboratory) has been involved in the study of mechanisms and methods of prevention of spread of infection for many years and this book describes the results of many studies made by the laboratory. It is hoped that it will provide readers with a greater understanding of why certain recommendations are made and help them to make decisions in new situations. Whenever possible decisions should be based on evidence and not conjecture. Clinical trials provide the most conclusive evidence but these are rarely possible; microbiological studies are preferred to arbitrary decisions based on opinions which maintain ritual methods.

Nevertheless, it is important to know whether a clinical problem exists and a knowledge of the incidence of infection is necessary. To introduce new control measures where there is no clinical problem is time-wasting and expensive, e.g. treating all foul linen as infected is of little value if laundry workers are never infected from foul linen, or the introduction of safety cabinets in haematology laboratories when laboratory-acquired hepatitis B is almost non-existent, and in any case does not spread in the air, is a pointless exercise.

This book does not contain a detailed account of control of infection methods and is complementary and not an alternative to 'Control of Hospital Infection: a Practical Handbook' (Ed. Lowbury, Ayliffe, Geddes and Williams) and to several excellent books published in the USA. Information on basic microbiology has been kept to a minimum and problems of administration have been mainly omitted as these topics are well covered elsewhere. Some references are included for further reading, but larger textbooks and particularly review articles in the 'Journal of Hospital Infection' and other journals should be referred to for more detailed information.

It is hoped that this book will be of particular value to the specialist Infection Control Nurse and microbiologist or Infection Control Officer, both during training and for subsequent reference. A knowledge of infection control is, however, increasingly required by other disciplines and is regularly included in training programmes and examinations. The authors are regularly asked to lecture or provide teaching material for the following disciplines: qualified nurses on specialist courses, e.g. intensive care, renal dialysis, operating theatre, nurse tutors, etc.; student nurses, medical students, trainee surgeons, laundry and domestic managers, CSSD, catering and engineering staff, also architects, supplies and environmental health officers. The varying needs of these groups were taken into consideration when compiling this book.

We wish to thank the staff of the Hospital Infection Research Laboratory, the many nurses, doctors and other hospital staff who collaborated in studies, Mrs J. E. Ayliffe for the Index, and particularly Mrs Barbara Homer for arranging and typing the material.

G.A.J.A.
B.J.C.
L.J.T.

# Contents

Chapter 1

# The control of hospital-acquired infection in the UK

A prevalence (cross-sectional) survey of 18 163 patients in 43 hospitals in the UK in 1980 showed that 19.1% were infected and of these 9.3% of the infections were hospital-acquired[1]. Of the hospital-acquired infections urinary tract infection was the most common (2.8%) followed by wound (1.7%), the lower respiratory tract (1.5%) and skin infections (1.2%). The organisms isolated are shown in Table 1.

**Table 1 Common organisms causing hospital-acquired infection**

|  | *Percentage* |
|---|---|
| *Staph. aureus* | 17.6 |
| *Strep. pneumoniae* | 1.8 |
| *E. coli* | 26.1 |
| *Proteus* spp. | 11.2 |
| *Klebsiella* spp. | 7.2 |
| *Ps. aeruginosa* | 7.0 |
| *H. influenzae* | 1.7 |
| *Bacteroides* spp. | 1.7 |
| *Candida* spp. | 4.1 |

Staphylococcal infections were still common, particularly in wounds, but acquired virus infections were rarely identified (0.8%). The prevalence study, in which all patients in a hospital are visited on one occasion only over a period of several weeks, tends to give a higher rate than an incidence study, which records infection as a percentage of total admissions or discharges over a defined period. The prevalence rate is higher since it incorporates length of stay, and infected patients tend to stay in longer. Prevalence rates carried out in other countries and in the West Midlands from 1968 to 1970 have also been about 10%[2]. Incidence studies of all hospital-acquired infection have rarely been made in the UK.

A study in a general hospital in Birmingham from 1971 to 1973 showed an incidence of 4.8% (total patients discharged 26 000). Of these, urinary tract infections were the most common (2%), followed by postoperative wound infections (1.1%); respiratory tract infections were 0.4% and other infections 1.3%. An incidence rate of about 5% has been frequently reported from other countries.

## The organization of infection control

As early as 1955 Colebrook recommended the appointment of full-time Infection Control Officers. The Cohen Committee (1959) supported this to some extent by suggesting that a senior member of the medical staff was appointed to carry out this function on a part-time basis, and in 1959 the first Infection Control Nurse was appointed by Dr Brendan Moore in Torbay. In the early 1960s hospitals began to organize Infection Control Committees and to appoint Infection Control Officers and Nurses. Infection control activities include the provision and implementation of infection control policies, surveillance, education, liaison with wards, theatres and departments, including laboratories, sterile services, occupational health, hotel services, etc.

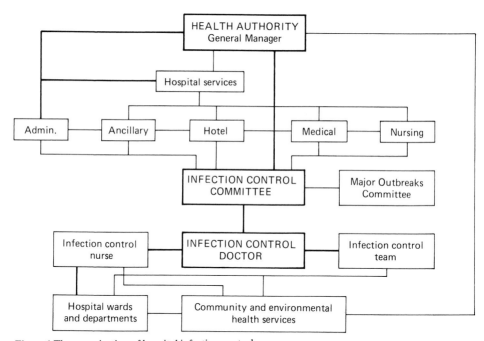

**Figure 1** The organization of hospital infection control

Although there are some variations, most large hospitals have the following committees or staff[3] (Figure 1).

1. Infection Control Committee (ICC).
2. Major Outbreaks Committee.
3. Infection Control Officer or Doctor (ICO or ICD).
4. Infection Control Nurse (ICN).
5. Infection Control Team (ICT).

The Infection Control Committee is responsible to the Health Authority through the General Manager for ensuring that policies exist to prevent the spread of infection in all areas of the hospital, e.g. policies for disinfection, isolation, aseptic techniques and use of antibiotics. This committee should also seek the authority and resources to implement agreed policy. The committee will usually consist of the Infection Control Officer (Doctor), Consultant Microbiologist, Infection Control Nurse, and the Medical Officer of Environmental Health (MOEH) as well as representatives of administration, medical, nursing, pharmacy, sterile services, and occupational health staff. Heads of other departments such as engineering, laundry, supplies and hotel services may either be permanent members or are invited to attend when their departments are being discussed. Representatives should be of sufficient seniority to be able to take some responsibility for the co-operation of their colleagues to ensure the implementation of agreed policy, and agenda should be circulated in sufficient time to allow adequate consultation. Committees are of varying size and meet at intervals ranging from monthly to annually, depending on the size of the hospital and occurrence of problems.

The Major Outbreaks Committee should be a standing committee called to assist when an outbreak occurs which requires the provision of additional or major redistribution of existing resources, or requires substantial changes in operational policy (see also pp. 30–31). The additional requirements may be for nursing, medical or ancillary staff or for supplies or services, e.g. laundry, disposable gloves, etc. Changes in policy may include the provision of additional isolation facilities, stopping admissions, closing specific wards, or restricting movements of patients or staff. The Committee should be convened by a senior administrator usually on the advice of the Infection Control Officer and should consist of:-

The Infection Control Officer*
A senior medical officer
The Infection Control Nurse
The Medical Officer of Environmental Health (if the infection is notifiable or likely to involve the community)
A senior administrator
A senior nurse
The Occupational Health Physician**
An infectious diseases physician**

Managers of hotel services or other departments may need to be co-opted if a special commitment is required during a specified outbreak, e.g. laundries in large outbreaks involving diarrhoea. The Infection Control Officer would normally co-ordinate investigations. Other functions of the committee should include all communications with the press, deciding on whether outside help is required and notifying other authorities if considered necessary, e.g. Regional Medical Officer, Department of Health, Communicable Diseases Surveillance Centre (CDSC) and other local hospitals. Good communications with the infected patient, their relatives and all staff involved are essential. Reassurance and explanation of the risk involved and the measures necessary to prevent spread should be given without an unnecessary breach of patient confidentiality.

The Infection Control Officer (Doctor) is responsible for the day-to-day implementation of infection control policy, and where infection problems outside

---

* The microbiologist and Chairman of the Infection Control Committee should be included if it is not the same person as the Infection Control Officer.
** Where appointed and if relevant to the type of infection.

existing policy arise, would normally be expected to take the necessary steps to prevent immediate spread pending a new policy being introduced by the committee. Medical staff have a high degree of clinical freedom and changes involving them are more likely to be made by persuasion rather than direction. The ICO should therefore be medically qualified and of sufficient seniority to influence his colleagues. Day-to-day contact and a knowledge of working conditions and problems within the hospital and some regular patient contact is important. Since infections have a microbiological aetiology and evaluating risk and assessing the required precautions and therapy involves an understanding of how microbes spread, function and survive in the environment and how they can be killed by disinfectants and antibiotics as well as their likely effect on people, the microbiologist is most likely to have the training and authority to carry out the task. The majority (over 80%) of ICOs are consultant microbiologists. If an appointment from another discipline is made, the ICO will need to work in close co-operation with the microbiologist particularly where investigations using laboratory facilities are involved.

Since improved collaboration for the control of infection between hospital and the community is required, a recent report* suggests a District Control of Infection Officer is appointed to co-ordinate their activities. The ICO would be the most suitable person for this responsibility.

The Infection Control Nurse is a registered nurse, usually with experience in surgery, paediatrics, intensive care, infectious diseases or other relevant specialities. Since ICNs are likely to be the only full-time infection control specialists and in regular contact with ward and departments, they should visit these areas frequently. Infection Control Nurses are responsible for ensuring that policies are known, understood and have a practical application. Where difficulties exist in the application of policy, or problems occur which are not covered by existing policy, this should be reported to the ICO so that changes can be made.

The nurses have a major advisory role, especially on nursing practices, also responsibilities for education of all staff and liaison between departments and surveillance of infection.

The Infection Control Team is responsible for the day-to-day investigation of problems and will usually investigate outbreaks and evaluate infection control methods and materials. The team may consist of the ICO, the ICN and often a Medical Laboratory Scientific Officer with a special interest in infection control. Representatives of other disciplines or areas may be co-opted to deal with specific problems.

## The cost of hospital-acquired infection

The true cost of hospital-acquired infection is largely unknown because it is made up of a large number of components. Individual components may be difficult to identify and their values unknown and difficult to calculate. However, these can be divided into the following groups: patients and their families, the community or state in general, and those affecting the individual hospitals.

*DHSS (1988) *Public Health in England. The Report of an Enquiry into the Future Development of the Public Health Function,* London, HMSO

## Costs to the patient and family

Loss of physical function and mental anguish may reduce activity and lead to loss of earnings and the cost of alternative labour in the home.

## Costs to the state

The state may lose tax from earned income or have to pay medical benefits. Capital costs to provide the additional facilities for the treatment of patients who would otherwise have been discharged will be increased.

## Costs to the hospital

*Direct costs*: increased use of dressings, pharmaceutical products including antibiotics, medical and nursing time and prolonged bed occupancy by patients.

*Indirect costs due to the presence of infection*: cost of microbiology, sterile supply, infection control services, operating theatres and isolation facilities.

Of these, the only cost that can be readily calculated is that of increased hospital stay. In England and Wales approximately 4.75 million patients are hospitalized every year and about 5% of these acquire an infection (237 500), and it can be assumed that on average an additional 4 days hospitalization results from the infection (950 000 additional bed days). The current cost of hospitalization for 1 day in an acute ward is approximately £120 per day. The total cost is therefore £114

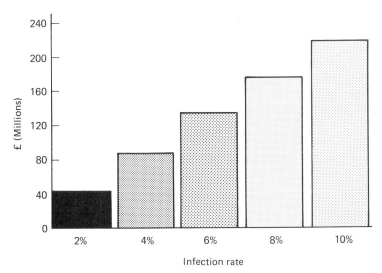

**Figure 2** Cost of infection in millions of pounds

million, and a potential saving of £22.8 million could be made for a 1% reduction in infection rate (Figure 2). The normal tendency would, however, be for infection rates to increase, since each year more high risk operations are carried out on an increasingly susceptible population. Maintaining existing infection rates would therefore be a substantial achievement.

## The cost-saving potential of infection control

There are very few full-time hospital appointments in infection control; approximately 200 full-time Infection Control Nurses or the equivalent at about £12 000 per year costs approximately £2.4 million. The Infection Research Laboratory in Birmingham and the Division of Hospital Infection are the only two full-time organizations devoted to research into infection control and both are small.

A study in the USA suggests that one Infection Control Nurse for every 250 beds and a physician with a specialist interest in infection control can reduce hospital-acquired infection by as much as 30%, and without such a service an increase of 18% could be expected over the same period[4]. While some infection control measures will undoubtedly cost money, research into evaluating measures can make large savings. A potential reduction of 30% may be expected or, even assuming that some hospitals already have a more effective programme, a 10% reduction may be obtainable. As a result of studies on the mechanisms and effectiveness of disinfecting environmental surfaces, a substantial reduction in the use of disinfectants has occurred without any measurable increase in infection rates. Research showing that wearing caps, masks and gowns and using ventilated dressing stations for dressing postoperative wounds did not reduce wound infection rates has probably allowed similar savings to be made over the same period. There is obviously a need to identify those methods most likely to be effective and to target them more precisely. The identification of unnecessary measures may still allow substantial savings to be made. However, it must be appreciated that the selection of priorities for controlling infection is not entirely within the hospital control. External pressures from Environmental Health Officers and the Health and Safety Executive can enforce expensive changes that are not always based on sound evidence or take into account other patient care priorities.

A scientific, or at least logical, explanation of how the proposed measures will reduce infection risk should be required. A reduction of the numbers of microbes present in the environment may not be sufficient explanation where there is no evidence that the existing level has caused infections. It should be appreciated that changes are likely to be motivated by the publicity given to risks newly perceived by outside groups or by groups with a special interest in improving their own area or image. Wherever possible resources should be allocated on scientifically evaluated assessment and should be specifically targeted at the method of spread. The fear of HIV infection has undoubtedly led to the introduction of irrational and expensive measures, e.g. the extensive introduction of surface disinfection when there is no evidence of infection acquired from non-penetrative surfaces and excessive use of disposable gloves in low risk populations.

Chapter 2

# Micro-organisms and their properties

A micro-organism or microbe is a rather loose term for any plant or animal which cannot be seen without a microscope and does not form organized tissues as do higher plants and animals. They are usually single-celled but some organisms, particularly fungi, are more complex. Micro-organisms causing disease in man may be divided into four groups – bacteria, viruses, fungi and protozoa.

## Bacteria

Bacteria are the main causes of hospital-acquired infection although viruses may occasionally cause an epidemic, particularly in children's wards. Bacteria are single-celled and are measured in microns ($\mu$m, i.e. 0.001 mm). They are variable in size and shape (Figure 3); bacilli are rod-shaped 2–5 mm × 0.8 mm in diameter; cocci are 0.8–1 mm and may exist in pairs (diplococci), bunches (staphylococci) or chains (streptococci). Others may exist as curved rods (vibrios) or spirals (spirochaetes). Bacteria may have other structures, such as filaments or flagella, which enable them to move in fluids, or a mucoid layer or capsule which protects some organisms, e.g. *Streptococcus pneumoniae* or *Klebsiella pneumoniae*, from the body defence mechanisms. Thick-walled structures (spores) may increase the resistance of certain bacteria, e.g. *Clostridium tetani, Clostridium welchii (perfringens)* and *Bacillus subtilis,* to moderate degrees of heat or to chemical disinfectants.

Bacteria usually multiply by binary fission, i.e. each organism increases in size, and then divides into two daughter cells. Other mechanisms of transferring genetic material may occur. In conjugation, two cells come together and genetic material (extrachromosomal) in a plasmid passes from one to another along a hollow tube or pilus. Conjugation is particularly important as resistance to antibiotics may be transferred by this method. Other methods of transfer of genetic material may take place, e.g. by a bacteriophage (transduction) or in deoxyribonucleic acid (DNA) from disrupted cells (transformation).

Bacteria are found everywhere – in the air, in soil and water – and few are pathogenic (capable of producing disease in man). They are present in the normal flora of the skin, in the mouth, vagina and the gastrointestinal tract. Organisms found on the skin are mainly *Staphylococcus epidermidis*, micrococci and diphtheroids (aerobic and anaerobic). *Streptococcus viridans, Branhamella*

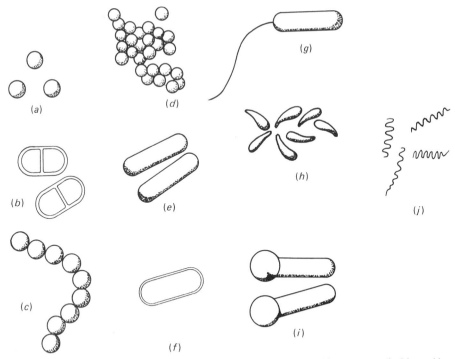

**Figure 3** Common bacterial forms: (a) coccus; (b) capsulated diplococci (pneumococci); (c) cocci in chains (streptococci); (d) cocci in clusters (staphylococci); (e) bacillus; (f) capsulated bacillus (e.g. *Klebsiella* spp.); (g) bacillus with polar flagellum (e.g. *Pseudomonas* spp.); (h) curved bacilli (e.g. *Vibrio* spp.); (i) spore-bearing bacillus (e.g. *Clostridium* spp.); (j) spiral bacillus (spirochaetes)

*catarrhalis* and anaerobic bacilli are found normally in the mouth and throat. *Escherichia coli, Proteus mirabilis, Klebsiella aerogenes, Streptococcus faecalis,* anaerobic Gram-negative bacilli (*Bacteroides*) are found in the lower intestinal tract. The organisms of the normal flora do not usually cause disease in the sites where they normally exist and tend to protect the host from other organisms. However, they may cause infection in other sites, e.g. *E. coli* in the urinary tract, *Strep. viridans* or *Staph. epidermidis* in subacute endocarditis, and *Bacteroides* may cause wound infection after operations on the colon or rectum.

Bacteria can be initially classified by their staining reaction. The Gram stain is the most useful. Gram-positive organisms stain a purplish-blue and include streptococci, staphylococci, aerobic and anaerobic sporing bacilli, e.g. *B. subtilis* and *Cl. welchii* or *Cl. tetani*. Gram-negative organisms stain red and include some cocci, *Neisseria gonorrhoeae, N. meningitidis,* most of the aerobic bacilli, e.g. *E. coli, Klebsiella,* and anaerobic non-sporing bacilli. Some organisms, such as *Mycobacterium tuberculosis,* may be identified by a special stain. Mycobacteria are acid-fast and show as red bacilli on a blue or green background in a Ziehl–Neelsen stain. *Corynebacterium diphtheriae* show granules on staining by Albert's or Neisser's stain.

Direct staining of specimens is of limited value, but may sometimes assist in the immediate diagnosis and treatment. Staphylococci or pneumococci may be recognized in purulent sputum and this may assist in the rapid diagnosis of pneumonia. Staphylococci in large numbers in the faeces suggest staphylococcal enteritis in a patient with severe diarrhoea. A direct film may be useful in diagnosing a urinary tract infection but is of little value for making decisions on the choice of an antibiotic.

The sample, e.g. swab, pus, urine, etc., is cultured on a plate (petri dish) containing artificial media. The medium is basically a nutrient broth solidified if necessary by a gelatin-like substance – agar. The nutrient broth provides protein, carbohydrate, essential salts and other factors at a pH suitable for bacterial growth. Most bacteria isolated from human beings or animals either require blood for their growth, or show an improved growth on blood-containing media. A blood-agar plate, nutrient broth with agar and horse-blood, is commonly used and haemolysis of the blood can help in recognition of the organisms. When the plate is incubated at 37°C for 18–24 hours bacteria grow as colonies, each containing millions of organisms. Other types of media are used, MacConkey medium (bile-salt lactose

**Table 2 Organisms and infections**

| Organisms | Infection | Main characteristics |
|---|---|---|
| Gram-positive | | |
| *Staphylococcus aureus* | Boils, wounds, osteomyelitis, food poisoning | Coagulase-positive, usually resistant to benzylpenicillin |
| *Staphylococcus epidermidis* | Intravenous sites, endocarditis, wounds | Coagulase-negative |
| *Streptococcus pyogenes* (Group A) | Tonsillitis, scarlet fever, burns and puerperal infection | Clear beta-haemolysis on blood agar, sensitive to benzylpenicillin |
| *Streptococcus faecalis* | Urinary tract, subacute endocarditis | Usually sensitive to ampicillin (not benzylpenicillin) |
| *Clostridium perfringens* | Gas gangrene, food poisoning | Anaerobic sporing bacillus, sensitive to benzylpenicillin |
| *Clostridium tetani* | Tetanus | Anaerobic, drum-stick spores, usually sensitive to benzylpenicillin |
| Gram-negative | | |
| *Escherichia coli* | Urinary tract, wounds, pelvic sepsis | LF, usually sensitive to commonly used antibiotics |
| *Klebsiella* spp. | Urinary tract, wounds respiratory tract | LF, ampicillin-resistant |
| *Proteus mirabilis* | Urinary tract, wounds | NLF, typical smell, resistant to tetracycline and nitrofurantoin |
| *Pseudomonas aeruginosa* | Wounds, burns, urinary tract, chest | NLF, typical smell, green pigment |
| *Salmonella* spp. | Enteric fever, food poisoning | NLF, motile |
| *Shigella* spp. | Dysentery | NLF, non-motile |
| *Campylobacter* spp. | Diarrhoea | NLF, (vibrio) |
| *Acinetobacter anitratus* | Urinary tract, wounds, respiratory tract | NLF, often resistant to usual antibiotics |
| *Serratia marcescens* | Urinary tract, wounds, respiratory tract | NLF, often red colonies, usually resistant to cephalosporins |
| *Legionella pneumophila* | Respiratory tract | Requires special media |
| *Bacteroides* spp. | Wounds, pelvic sepsis, lung abscess | Anaerobic, non-sporing |

LF, lactose fermenter; NLF, non-lactose fermenter.

agar) is useful for intestinal organisms. Other media are selective for pathogens, e.g. deoxycholate–citrate agar, for isolation of salmonellae or shigellae from faeces. In recent years anaerobes have increased in importance and are recognized by growth on plates incubated in the absence of oxygen.

Further tests may be necessary to identify organisms and include biochemical, e.g. fermentation of sugars, and serological to identify specific strains of salmonella or shigella. Antibiotic sensitivity tests may sometimes assist in identification.

The common organisms causing hospital infection and their properties are shown in Table 2.

The growth of bacteria in solutions is relevant to many problems in hospital infection. Typically in nutrient broth, there is a latent period lasting for 2–4 hours in which no growth occurs, followed by a logarithmic phase, a stationary phase, and later a phase of decline when the organisms begin to die (Figure 4).

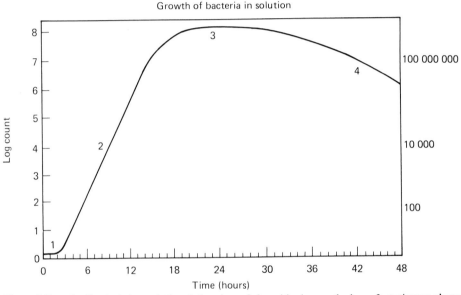

**Figure 4** Growth of bacteria in a solution: 1, lag phase; 2, logarithmic growth phase; 3, stationary phase; 4, decline phase

A similar growth pattern may be seen in urine and demonstrates the reason for examining urines within 2–3 hours before growth occurs. Refrigeration at 4°C will prevent the organism from growing. Similar principles apply to the growth of bacteria in food which should be stored at temperatures below 4°C or above 65°C. Most bacteria fail to grow above 50°C except for some thermophilic strains, e.g. *Bacillus stearothermophilus*, which are non-pathogenic. The growth cycle described occurs in optimal conditions of temperature and nutrients and for most human pathogens this is between 35°C and 38°C. However, growth may be observed at lower temperatures (e.g. 20–25°C) but may take several days to reach the stationary phase. Some organisms, particularly *Klebsiella* and *Enterobacter,* are able to grow in the environment and may reach large numbers in 24 hours with minimal nutrients. *Pseudomonas aeruginosa* can also grow to large numbers at room temperature in 24–48 hours in distilled water. This explains the heavy growth of this organism obtained in washing bowls, shaving brushes, humidifiers, mops or endoscopes, which have not been adequately disinfected or dried. Other pseudomonads are able to grow in weak disinfectant solutions and have been reported in solutions of quaternary ammonium compounds, chlorhexidine, hexachlorophane, and occasionally in phenolics.

Gram-negative bacilli can often adapt themselves to grow in concentrations of disinfectant which would normally kill them in laboratory tests. This is likely if solutions are topped-up when the container is empty instead of cleaning it and completely replacing with a new solution. This tends to occur with handwashing soaps or disinfectant solutions unless a suitable preservative is added. Contamination of tanks of disinfectant used for urine bottles has been reported because of topping-up rather than replacing the disinfectant solution. Dilute solutions of disinfectants are also often unstable.

Bacteria vary in their ability to grow in fluids. Staphylococci fail to grow in dextrose–saline at room temperature whereas *Klebsiella* and *Serratia* grow well. The risks of infection from intravenous fluids are much greater with these Gram-negative bacilli than with most other potential pathogens such as staphylococci, *E. coli,* etc. which require a higher temperature and additional nutrients to grow properly. Airborne organisms from the skin, coagulase-negative staphylococci, are only likely to get into intravenous fluids in small numbers when a container is opened for the addition of other fluids and are unlikely to grow. Greater care is necessary with intravenous alimentation therapy as sufficient

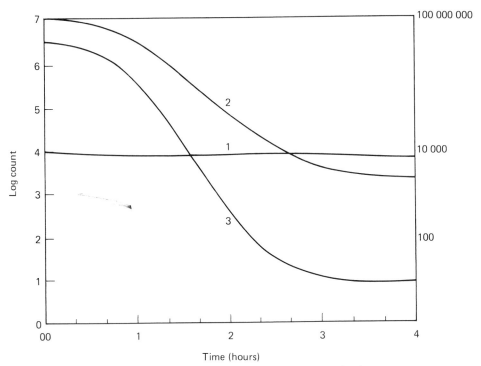

**Figure 5** Survival of organisms on drying. Suspensions of organisms allowed to dry at room temperature over 4 hours. 1, Spores survive well; 2, *Staph. aureus* shows moderate survival; 3, *Ps. aeruginsoa* (and other Gram-negative bacilli) rapidly die on drying

nutrient is available for other organisms, such as *Candida,* to grow; additions to these fluids should be made in a ventilated cabinet in the pharmacy, unless the fluid is used within a few hours.

Although some Gram-negative bacilli can grow in fluids with minimal nutrients at room temperature, they are very susceptible to drying. *E. coli, Pseudomonas, Klebsiella,* and some other organisms, such as *Candida,* die rapidly on drying (Figure 5), but staphylococci show greater survival[5]. The implications are that Gram-negative bacilli rarely spread in the air, unless in an aerosol, whereas the airborne route is a mode of spread for staphylococci. Nevertheless, staphylococci die on dry surfaces over several days and even after overnight the numbers are considerably reduced[6]. The risks of transfer from the inanimate environment are small even though some cells survive for months. Spore-bearing bacilli also survive well in the dry environment but are mostly non-pathogenic, e.g. *B. subtilis.* Clostridia are commonly isolated in the dry environment of the hospital, usually in small numbers, but rarely cause a problem. Beta-haemolytic streptococci survive poorly on drying, but large numbers have been found on blankets and in dust during outbreaks of infection. However, in recent years environmental contamination has not been apparent in our experience.

A small number of Gram-negative bacilli will survive drying if the initial number of organisms is large, and they are protected by organic matter. This explains why *Ps. aeruginosa* can often be isolated from floors in burns units and possibly why airborne spread of enteropathogenic *E. coli* or *Salmonella* has occasionally been reported. Some Gram-negative bacilli, e.g. epidemic strains of *Klebsiella* and *Acinetobacter anitratus* survive drying better than others. This may have epidemiological significance by improving their chance of spread in the hands. From the evidence available, thorough washing and drying is the best method of reducing any small risks of spread from the dry environment. Storing nail-brushes and thermometers in fluids has always been a potential hazard, particularly if fresh solutions are not made up daily. Common source outbreaks of *Pseudomonas* infection are now much less common since equipment is more often stored in a dry state. The relevance of these properties to the spread of infection will be considered in a later chapter.

## Viruses

Viruses are small infective particles 20–200 nm in size (1000 nm = 1 mm, which is the size of a staphylococcal cell) and can only grow in living cells. Viral disease is diagnosed by growing in tissue cultures or by serological tests. Monoclonal antibodies are increasingly being used for rapid diagnosis of viral infections, e.g. by immunofluorescence. The survival of viruses in the environment is generally poor, and close contact is usually necessary for transmission. However, if large numbers are dispersed some will survive for relatively long periods. Hepatitis B virus (HBV) will survive for up to 7 days. Human immunodeficiency virus (HIV), a retrovirus causing AIDS, will survive for several days, but is readily killed by most disinfectants. Viruses are not a major cause of endemic infection in hospital but outbreaks of childhood viral infections (e.g. respiratory syncytial virus) can cause problems in paediatric wards. Some viruses, such as herpes simplex or zoster and cytomegalovirus, are particularly hazardous in immunosuppressed patients.

# Fungi

These are more complex structures than bacteria and may grow as filaments (mycelia) and produce reproductive spores. They can be grown on inanimate culture media, such as Sabouraud's. They are identified by their microscopic appearance, colonial morphology and sometimes by biochemical and serological tests. *Candida albicans* is the commonest fungus causing infection in hospital and may spread in neonatal units. It usually infects debilitated patients. Other fungi may cause infection in hospital but mostly in immunosuppressed patients. *Aspergillus fumigatus* is an example. Other fungi are rare, e.g. *Cryptococcus neoformans* may sometimes be found in the compromised host. Aspergilli are common airborne contaminants and possibly isolating the compromised patient in a room with filtered air may reduce the likelihood of infection. *Cr. neoformans* is found in bird droppings but whether this is a source of infection in hospital is uncertain.

# Protozoa

Protozoa are single-celled members of the animal kingdom and are rarely a cause of hospital infection. It is possible that malaria could be transferred in transfused blood but is very rare in Northern Europe and the USA. *Entamoeba histolytica*, a causative organism of dysentery, is also not readily directly transferred from person to person in hospital. Other protozoa tend to be found mainly in the compromised host, but the infections are usually present and are re-activated due to immunological incompetence. *Pneumocystis carinii, Toxoplasma gondii, Giardia lamblia* and cryptosporidia are examples of protozoa occurring in these patients.

# Laboratory testing of microbiology specimens

Laboratory tests are time-consuming and expensive and unnecessary tests should be avoided. Common reasons for wastage of resources are: unsuitable or unnecessary specimens, inadequate information on laboratory request forms, reports of little or doubtful value to the clinician.

### Collection of specimens

Pus should be sent to the laboratory whenever available; swabs taken from the pus are of less value. Many organisms, e.g. β-haemolytic streptococci, die rapidly on dry swabs. Pus or swabs in transport media should be sent to the laboratory as soon as possible if anaerobic culture is required. Sometimes the laboratory will supply special containers.

'Sputum' consisting of saliva only is useless and reports are misleading. Urine is a good culture medium and should be sent to the laboratory or refrigerated within 2 hours of collection. Dip-slides may be preferable if rapid delivery to the laboratory or refrigeration is not possible. CSF and other fluids should be delivered as soon as possible to the laboratory as cells tend to disintegrate rapidly and delicate pathogens, e.g. *N. meningitidis*, may die. Samples of faeces are preferable to rectal swabs, but if swabs are taken they should show the presence of faeces; anal swabs (instead of rectal) are usually useless and may be misleading.

Containers for specimens should be filled aseptically to avoid contamination from organisms on the outside of the container, also to prevent contamination of the outside from organisms in the specimen. False outbreaks of infection have occurred due to collection of samples from several patients in an unsterile container, e.g. urine in a bowl or jug, before transfer to the sterile laboratory container.

Viruses survive poorly on dry swabs and samples (swabs and washings) should be collected in special transport media and taken to the laboratory as soon as possible. If in doubt consult the laboratory; often laboratory personnel will prefer to collect their own specimens. Many virus infections can only be diagnosed serologically; blood from acute and convalescent stages of disease is required to demonstrate at least a four-fold rise in antibody titre.

It is most important that samples are taken before treatment is started. If septicaemia is suspected two or more blood cultures should be taken at short intervals between them; treatment need not be delayed beyond 30 minutes.

Samples should also be correctly taken. Nose swabs should be moistened in sterile saline and rubbed several times firmly around each of the anterior nares. Throat swabs should be taken from the inflamed area, preferably obtaining some exudate. Contamination with saliva should be avoided. Careful cleaning of the vulva is necessary when collecting a mid-stream specimen of urine from a female. In general, superficial contamination should be avoided when collecting samples from infected lesions. Occasionally invasive techniques are necessary to obtain adequate or non-contaminated specimens, e.g. transtracheal aspiration, suprapubic puncture, aspiration of abscess.

Specimens should only be sent if the results are likely to provide or confirm a diagnosis or exclude a likely diagnosis. Routine screening is rarely a cost-effective exercise and if undertaken should only be carried out in consultation with the microbiologist. All routine screening programmes should be checked at intervals of not more than 3 months. This will often show that either sufficient evidence is already available or that positive tests are so rare that continuation cannot be justified on cost alone or that treatment can be decided by alternative means.

When doubt exists the laboratory should always be consulted so that the most suitable specimen and method of collection can be agreed, and that the needs of the patient and priorities of the laboratory can be taken into consideration. All specimens are put through a routine procedure which will not always provide the answer to a specific problem. The microbiologist should be consulted about any problem patient.

**Inadequate information on request forms**

Forms should be carefully designed so that the required information is likely to be provided by the clinician. The following information is necessary:

1. Age of patient: host susceptibility and diseases vary with age, e.g. enteropathogenic *E. coli* may be relevant in young infants but not adults.
2. Name and number: the patient's hospital number should always be included. Names are often the same and mistakes can occur.

3. Ward: this is needed so that infection control staff can detect outbreaks, as well as ensuring the report is returned without delay.
4. Relevant history: this is most important as tests may be decided on this. A swab from a patient with puerperal sepsis is treated differently from one with a vaginal discharge. Writing 'wound swab' may waste time if it is really from a pressure sore. The cause of infection might be anaerobic and a suitable culture might not be made.
5. Site of infection: different areas of the body tend to have their own flora and the same organisms elsewhere may have a pathogenic role. *Staph. aureus* may be a normal inhabitant of the nose, but not in an infected finger.
6. Antibiotic therapy: failure to include this information often leads to a misleading report. The antibiotic may inhibit growth of the causative organism or select resistant strains which colonize the site, e.g. ampicillin-resistant klebsiellas are common in sputa of patients treated with ampicillin but rarely are a cause of clinical lung disease.
7. Date and time of collection: different organisms survive for varying periods and some grow well at room temperature. Sputa left overnight may show a heavy growth of *Candida* which is not significant. Even if a swab is placed in transport medium some Gram-negative bacilli may grow over several days.

## Environmental sampling

Bacteria are normally present, often in large numbers, in an occupied environment. The types and numbers of organisms depend on the number of people occupying the area and their activity, the proportion of each sex present, the flow of air and the humidity. Bacterial counts of the air can change rapidly depending on circumstances. In general, the patient is much more likely to contaminate the environment than to be infected by it. For these reasons environmental sampling is of limited value.

Routine sampling of air and surfaces in operating theatres, wards, catering areas and pharmacies is unnecessary. If a sampling programme is agreed it should be justified and have a specific objective; possible reasons are:

1. To identify routes of spread of infection.
2. To identify staphylococcal dispersers.
3. To evaluate cleaning or disinfection techniques, usually for research or teaching purposes.

When such procedures are required the microbiologist should be consulted as interpretation requires experience in this field.

### Sampling techniques

Swabbing of surfaces, unless taken from a defined area using a standard technique, will indicate only the presence or absence of a limited range of organisms. Growth of *Cl. welchii* from a broth culture of a swab taken from the floor of an operating theatre is no reason for closing the theatre suite.

Contact plates give a semi-quantitative result and are useful for comparing surfaces and also indicate the distribution of organisms on the surface. The technique is useful for detecting the presence of a staphylococcal disperser and large numbers of samples can be rapidly taken from surfaces. Separate plates are, of course, necessary for aerobic and anaerobic organisms. Contact plates are unsuitable for counting very large numbers of organisms and may show a semi-confluent or confluent growth. Washings from a defined area of a surface remove more organisms, and also tend to break up clumps, giving much higher counts than contact plates. More accurate counts are obtained especially with large numbers of organisms, but give no indication of spatial arrangement.

Air samples are usually measured with a slit sampler or by exposing settle plates. The slit sampler demonstrates the number of colony-forming units in the air, but many may be small particles which would not fall into a wound. Sizes of bacteria-carrying particles can be measured with an Anderson or a Cascade sampler. A useful portable air sampler is now available[7].

Settle plates measure the bacteria-carrying particles falling onto the plate over a defined period but not the total numbers in the air. However, this is a simple technique and is useful for identifying staphylococcal dispersers in a ward or theatre.

Fluids should be sampled with a pipette and total organisms counted. It is important that whenever the environment is sampled, the technique used should be quantitative or semi-quantitative if any useful conclusions are to be made from the observations.

## Typing of bacteria

Most infections acquired in hospital are caused by organisms which are part of the normal flora, e.g. *Staph. aureus* or *E. coli*, or are commonly found in the environment, e.g. *Kl. aerogenes* or *Ps. aeruginosa*.

*Ps. aeruginosa* can be found in 25% or more of hospital sinks but these strains are usually of different types from those causing infections[8]. *Staph. aureus* is present in the noses of 20% of healthy people and typing studies have shown that strains isolated from ward nurses rarely cause wound infections. The identification of the species in these instances is rarely of value. It therefore may be necessary to use additional methods, e.g. typing, to establish whether strains have originated from a single source or are epidemiologically related. On the other hand, the isolation of an unusual organism, such as *S. typhi*, from two or more patients in a ward is highly suggestive of cross-infection without the necessity of additional typing methods.

The following typing methods are commonly used – biotyping, antibiograms and resistograms, serological, phage or bacteriocin.

### Biotyping

This method is an extension of the biochemical techniques commonly used for identification of species, i.e. enzyme production, fermentation of sugars, as already described. It is of limited value in the subdivision of species, but may be useful for characterizing organisms such as *Acinetobacter* spp. or even *E. coli* where other typing methods are not routinely available in a routine laboratory. A wide range of tests is usually necessary, e.g. over 20, making this a rather expensive method. Occasionally a strain may have an unusual property, such as an indole-positive *Klebsiella*, which enables it to be sufficiently well characterized for epidemiological purposes in an outbreak in one ward, but not as a general typing method.

## Antibiograms and resistograms

Antibiograms are usually not very helpful as many strains show similar patterns. Most staphylococcal wound infections are caused by strains resistant to penicillin only and *Kl. aerogenes* tends to be resistant to the common antibiotics, but differences between strains are often not sufficient to characterize individual strains. However, some strains of *Staph. aureus* or Gram-negative bacilli are resistant to four or five antibiotics and this may be sufficient to identify a strain in a ward. It is likely that strains of *Staph. aureus* resistant to methicillin, gentamicin, erythromycin and tetracycline isolated from several patients in a ward are the same strain. Occasionally resistance to a single antibiotic may be equally useful. Gentamicin resistance in *Ps. aeruginosa* may be sufficient evidence to suggest a single strain is spreading in a unit, but is not entirely reliable. Antibiotic resistance is usually controlled by a plasmid, which can be transferred between genera as well as species and plasmids can be lost so that antibiograms must be used with caution in identifying single strains. Nevertheless, the method is one of the most useful in routine laboratories.

Resistograms are similar to antibiograms except sensitivity is measured to a range of chemicals. Although this method is useful for typing organisms, such as *E. coli*, *Proteus* or *Candida* for which other methods are not readily available, it is difficult to control. Most laboratories could use this method, but the requirement is so rare that it is not usually worth setting it up as a routine procedure.

## Serological typing

This method is commonly used for routinely identifying species, particularly *Salmonella* and *Shigella*. Since more than one strain, e.g. *Salmonella typhimurium*, is not likely to be in a ward at the same time, identification other than of the species is usually sufficient. Additional typing may be necessary in the community where it may be useful to determine the source of a strain of *Salmonella*, e.g. in an outbreak of food poisoning where animals or a certain farm is suspect. However, serological typing of commonly isolated strains such as *Klebsiella* and *Ps. aeruginosa* can be of considerable value in investigating outbreaks of hospital infection. Serological types are usually stable, but sometimes serotyping must be combined with other methods, such as phage or bacteriocin, as some serotypes are particularly common.

## Phage typing[9]

Phages are small virus-like particles which grow in bacterial cells and usually destroy them. A typical phage is shown in Figure 6. It consists of a head containing deoxyribonucleic acid (DNA) and a tail. The hollow tail attaches itself to the bacterial wall and DNA passes along it into the bacterial cells. The phage DNA takes over the DNA-producing mechanism of the bacterial cell and makes more phage. The cell is destroyed and this is known as lysis. Phage particles escape and enter and destroy other cells. A drop of phage concentrate on a plate seeded with sensitive bacteria and incubated will show a clear area of lysis.

Phages tend to be active against certain bacterial strains and if a number of different phages are used a pattern of lysis is obtained (Figure 7). Staphylococcal phage typing is the commonest method used in hospitals. A set of numbered phage suspensions are applied to plates seeded with unknown types of *Staph. aureus* and

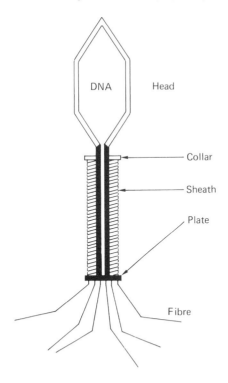

DNA    Head

Collar

Sheath

Plate

Fibre

**Figure 6** Diagram of phage

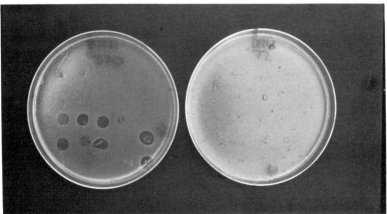

**Figure 7** Phage typing of *Staph. aureus*

after overnight incubation the pattern of lysis is read. Staphylococcal phages are divided into three groups and numbered as shown below in Table 3. Group I strains, e.g. 52/80, 29/52A/80, are commonly found in normal noses and can cause boils and septic lesions. Group II strains, especially 71, may cause impetigo. Group III strains, e.g. 6/47 53/54/75, may cause wound infections. However, all phage types can be found in the noses of healthy people.

Phage types are considered to be different if there are two major differences, especially if different groups are involved, e.g. 52 is different from 52/52A/79.

**Table 3 Staphylococcal phages**

| Group I | 29 | 52 | 52A | 79 | 80 | (81) | |
|---|---|---|---|---|---|---|---|
| Group II | 3A | 3C | 55 | 71 | | | |
| Group III | 6 | 42E | 47 | 51 | 54 | 75 | 77 |
| | 83A | 84 | 85 | | | | |
| Miscellaneous | 94 | 95 | 96 | 88 | | | |

It must be realized that phage typing shows differences but similar types are not necessarily related. It is unlikely that a strain 52 isolated in the USA will be related epidemiologically to a similar type isolated in the UK.

### Bacteriocins

These are antibiotic-like substances produced by bacteria. As with phages, they are specific to species and usually to strains. Tests are made by growing the unknown strain on a culture plate and recording the inhibition of indicator strains (Figure 8). Patterns of inhibition are recorded as in phage typing. The method is useful for typing *Ps. aeruginosa*[10] or *Klebsiella,* but is often insufficiently discriminatory unless combined with another method.

### Other methods

New methods of typing have recently been described, e.g. plasmid and polypeptide profiles, DNA probes, and will be increasingly used in the future.

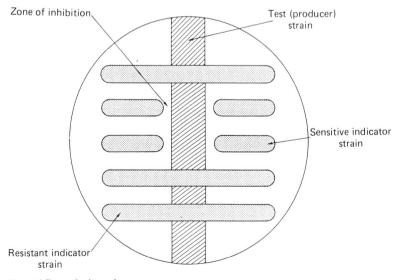

**Figure 8** Bacteriocin typing

Chapter 3

# Infection and the spread of micro-organisms

## Infection

Infection means the deposition of organisms in tissues and their growth with an associated host reaction. If the response of the host is slight or nil, this is usually termed 'colonization'. An example is the acquisition of a strain of *Staphylococcus aureus* in the nose of a healthy person. The staphylococcus grows in the anterior nares without causing any tissue reaction and the person is unaware of being a carrier. Organisms colonize other body sites, e.g. coagulase-negative cocci (*Staphylococcus epidermidis*) grow on normal skin, and *Escherichia coli* is a normal inhabitant of the intestinal tract. *Staph. aureus* and various Gram-negative bacilli are often found on the surface of operation wounds, varicose ulcers or pressure sores without apparently causing any additional tissue damage. Growth of organisms associated with a tissue reaction (i.e. inflammation) is usually referred to as sepsis or clinical infection. A septic wound is usually hot, red and swollen and will eventually produce pus, and bacteriological culture will usually show a heavy growth of the causative organism. A colonized wound may produce a similar growth but the wound will look healthy. For this reason, a wound or other lesion should not be called infected unless there is evidence of tissue damage. Nevertheless, colonization may be an important indication of an organism spreading in a ward or unit.

### How many organisms are required to cause an infection?

Another major problem is defining an infective dose. Large numbers of *Staph. aureus*, e.g. 100 000 cells ($10^5$) can be applied to the intact skin without causing a clinical infection and even if this number is injected, an infection may not necessarily occur. However, in the presence of a foreign body, such as a suture, 100 ($10^2$) organisms may start a clinical infection[11]. Small numbers of organisms may cause infection if they are able to grow without interference by the body's defences, e.g. in a haematoma. Similarly, large numbers of salmonella may be ingested without infection, but if gastric acidity is deficient infection may be caused by small numbers.

The susceptibility of the host is of major importance and this can rarely be assessed. Factors such as age, sex, pre-existing disease may all be of importance, but are difficult to quantify in terms of susceptibility in an individual. Deficiencies in defence mechanisms can rarely be detected in routine tests.

Another unknown variable is the virulence of the organism; unfortunately no laboratory test is available to determine differences in virulence between strains of the organisms usually causing hospital infection.

For infection to occur organisms from a source or reservoir must reach a susceptible site in sufficient numbers, which are difficult to define. Should disinfection of the hands or a surface reduce potential pathogens to less than 1000, 100, 10 or to nil? The hands are more important than the floor, as they are more likely to transfer organisms to a susceptible site. For practical purposes it would seem advisable to reduce potential pathogenic organisms on the hands to less than 100 or on a surface to less than 1000. Although it might seem desirable to reduce them to nil, this may require much more effort and be unnecessary to prevent the spread of infection. Removal of all potential pathogens from the skin of an operation site is obviously desirable, but the necessity of removing the normal flora remains uncertain except possibly in certain high risk operations.

Numbers of organisms in the environment are discussed in later chapters. Removal of all organisms from instruments is obviously much easier than from skin. Nevertheless, numbers on surfaces well away from the patient, e.g. on floors, are of minor relevance. A further problem is that organisms may be in clumps or otherwise protected. One skin scale containing 100 staphylococcal cells is more likely to initiate an infection than a scale containing 10, yet both will produce one colony on a settle plate. The distribution is also relevant, e.g. large numbers on the finger-tips are more important than a similar number on the back of the hand.

## The spread of micro-organisms

Micro-organisms commonly spread by the airborne route, or by direct or indirect contact. The mode of spread of infection in hospital is rarely certain but apart from

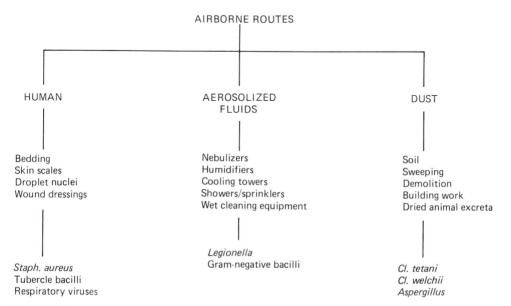

**Figure 9** Airborne spread

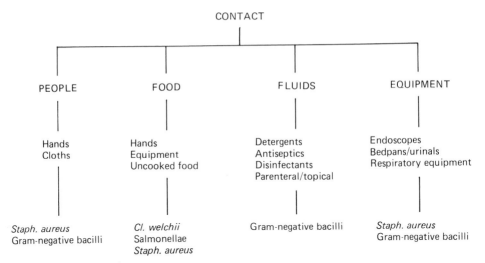

**Figure 10** Contact spread

respiratory viruses the airborne route is usually a minor one. Common modes of spread and organisms are shown in Figures 9 and 10 and are either endogenous or exogenous. Endogenous infections are acquired from the patient's own bacterial flora and exogenous from other patients or staff (cross-infection) or inanimate sources. In addition to contact and airborne routes, spread may occur by injection of parenteral fluids (Gram-negative bacilli) and blood (HBV and HIV).

The major factors in the spread of infection are: the numbers of organisms shed from the source, their ability to survive after leaving the source, their virulence, and the means of reaching a susceptible site on the same or another person in sufficient numbers to cause an infection. In this section we shall mainly consider the shedding of organisms and their survival. Heavy dispersal is one of the major factors.

**Staphylococcal infection**

This organism colonizes the anterior nares in about 20% of healthy individuals, occasionally the perineum and rarely other areas of skin. Other areas may be contaminated from a carrier site, e.g. the face, neck, hair and hands from a heavy nasal carrier, or the buttocks, abdomen and fingers from a perineal carrier (Figure 11). However, abnormal skin (e.g. eczematous) may be heavily colonized. Staphylococci are rarely shed directly into the air from the nose or mouth during normal breathing or talking, but are mainly shed on skin scales from areas of contaminated skin, e.g. the face or hands. This explains why masks are of little value in preventing the transfer of *Staph. aureus* from staff to patients. A person who sheds large numbers of *Staph. aureus* into the air is known as a disperser and is a particular danger in an operating theatre. Dispersers usually have large numbers of staphylococci on the carrier site, e.g. the nose or perineum, and the organisms tend to contaminate other areas of skin in greater numbers than carriers of small numbers.

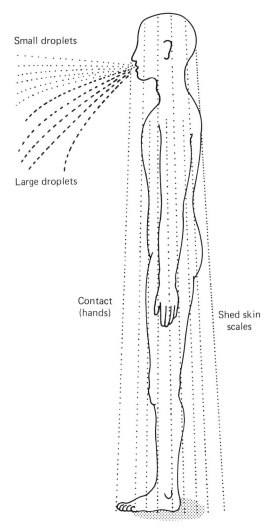

Small droplets

Large droplets

Contact
(hands)

Shed skin
scales

**Figure 11** Microbial dispersal

Dispersal is measured by air-sampling in a small room or plastic chamber while the person concerned carries out some standard exercises or removes clothes. Table 4 shows that healthy males tend to disperse more than healthy females, possibly because they shed more skin scales[12, 13]. Male perineal carriers tend to be dispersers and should be looked for in an outbreak in an operating theatre.

The additional risk of spread of *Staph. aureus* from long hair and beards is often queried. In general, these are only a hazard if the person is a heavy nasal or skin carrier of an epidemic strain. In our experience most of the outbreaks of theatre-acquired infection arise from staff with lesions, e.g. boils, eczema and fungal infections of the groin, although occasionally airborne spread will occur from healthy carriers. In the ward heavy dispersers are usually patients with discharging purulent lesions, bed sores, burns and widespread skin lesions; an

**Table 4 Dispersal of *Staphylococcus aureus* from nasal carriers**

| | | No. of colonies in 50 cu ft of air | | |
|---|---|---|---|---|
| | No. of subjects | 0–20 | 21–50 | >50 |
| Females | 30 | 29 (97%) | 1  (3%) | 0 |
| Males | 34 | 23 (67%) | 5 (15%) | 6 (18%) |

eczematous patient colonized with a potential epidemic strain in a surgical ward is a major hazard.

As already described, *Staph. aureus* survives well on drying and obviously spreads by the airborne route, but in the hospital the opportunities for spread by contact are as great or greater. A heavy disperser will contaminate clothing and bedding and will readily contaminate the hands and clothing of attendants. Organisms can be transferred to other patients in much greater numbers by contact than in the air. This demonstrates again that handwashing and wearing a protective plastic apron when in contact with an infected patient is much more important than an expensive ventilation system. It should also be remembered that although staphylococci survive fairly well in a dry environment, they do not grow and gradually die. Numbers of organisms shed into the dry environment decrease within a few days to small numbers, although some survive for months. Airborne contamination of fomites, e.g. curtains and furnishings, and of floors, plays a minor role in the spread of staphylococci and a room left overnight after occupation by a patient infected with staphylococci is unlikely to be responsible for infecting a subsequent patient. Nevertheless, it is still advisable to clean thoroughly a room after occupation by a heavy disperser of a virulent or epidemic strain.

Routine screening of staff is not of value since it is not possible to determine virulent or epidemic staphylococci from laboratory tests. However, epidemic strains are often resistant to several antibiotics and tend to occur in much larger numbers in the environment than the more sensitive non-epidemic strains. Much more rarely, sensitive or penicillin-resistant strains may spread if dispersed in large numbers, e.g. from a patient with a urinary tract infection, but rarely spread to many patients unless in a neonatal nursery. Endogenous spread of *Staph. aureus* from a carrier site to an operation or traumatic wound during surgery is a common mode of infection. How this occurs remains uncertain as staphylococci can rarely be found on or around the operation site after effective skin disinfection.

*Coagulase-negative staphylococci*
Coagulase-negative staphylococci are causing an increasing number of infections, particularly following implant surgery, in immunosuppressed patients and in neonates. Spread occurs as with *Staph. aureus*, but the organisms are present as residents on all areas of skin and are often more difficult to remove by disinfectants. Airborne spread has been shown to occur from staff in the operating room. Strains may be resistant to several antibiotics, often including gentamicin and methicillin. The difficulty of differentiating strains and the large number of different types found on normal skin make it difficult to define the mode of spread and whether infections are endogenous or exogenous, but epidemics appear to be rare.

## Gastrointestinal infections

These are spread from the faeces of an infected or colonized person or from contaminated food. In general, a heavy dose of organisms is required unless gastric acid is absent. During the acute stages of dysentery, infantile gastroenteritis caused by enteropathogenic *E. coli* or salmonellae, large numbers of organisms are shed in the faeces. In infants this may be associated with heavy environmental contamination. The organisms tend to die rapidly on drying, but if the initial numbers shed are very high some will survive and may even be transferred by the airborne route. This has been reported for enteropathogenic *E. coli* and salmonellae. However, this is rare and in our investigations, environmental sampling in rooms of infected patients have so far yielded few organisms except from bedding in immediate contact with the patient. In recent years, outbreaks of rotavirus infections have been increasingly reported in infant nurseries and in geriatric establishments. Large numbers of virus particles are found in the faeces and spread is again probably associated with heavy environmental contamination and dispersal.

Sometimes contaminated equipment has been responsible for the spread of enteropathogens, e.g. resuscitation equipment in neonates, but the main mode of spread is on the hands or possibly the clothing of attendants.

After the acute stages of diarrhoeal infections have passed, organisms in the faeces are less frequent and transmission is uncommon in adults. Infection can occur from carriers but provided care is taken with personal hygiene the risk is small. Spread from food is described in Chapter 14. *Clostridium difficile* causes pseudomembranous colitis and there is some evidence of spread in wards. The route remains uncertain, but transfer on sigmoidoscopes has been suggested.

## Other Gram-negative bacilli

Most infections caused by Gram-negative bacilli are endogenous in origin. Transfer is directly to the wound from the operation site in the intestinal tract or via the urethra to the urinary tract. Cross-infection is mainly on the hands of staff but spread can occur from contaminated equipment, e.g. wash bowls, urinals, bedpans, respiratory equipment. Since Gram-negative bacilli die rapidly on drying, airborne spread is rare. It has been reported from nebulizers contaminated with *Pseudomonas aeruginosa*. Spread by aerosols from contaminated cleaning equipment is a possibility, but reports of wounds infected from this source are unconvincing. Airborne spread is possible when burns dressings are changed. Presumably this is again an instance of dispersal of very large numbers of which some survive. Gram-negative bacilli can rarely be isolated in air of burns or intensive care wards and this mode of spread must be rare. *Acinetobacter anitratus* survives well in the environment and is sometimes part of the resident skin flora. It can spread in the air. *Legionella* is spread in aerosols from cooling towers and showers. Spread has also been reported from hot water systems.

## Respiratory infections

Viral infections involving the upper respiratory tract spread in the air as droplet nuclei, although recent evidence suggests that spread on the hands may be important. Influenza virus can survive for some hours on inanimate surfaces. It is likely that both airborne and contact play a role in the spread of these viruses. Heavy dispersers are again the main sources and cross-infection is most likely in the late incubation period or early days of an infection when virus concentrations are highest. As the concentration falls, the risks of transmission decrease. Some infections are particularly likely to spread in the air, e.g. chicken-pox and to a lesser extent measles. It is likely that the dose required to initiate infection in these diseases is low in susceptible individuals. Respiratory syncytial virus can spread in a paediatric unit, presumably in the air. Survival of respiratory viruses on surfaces in wards has been poorly evaluated. Herpes simplex virus will also survive on surfaces for several days but spread by this route is probably rare.

Tuberculosis is the other important infection which spreads in the air. The patient with an open lesion of the lung and large numbers of organisms in the sputum, i.e. the heavy disperser, is the main hazard. Spread from other types of tuberculosis, e.g. urinary tract, is unlikely as numbers tend to be smaller and the opportunity to reach a susceptible site in the respiratory tract of another person is minimal.

**Parenteral spread**

The problems of growth of organisms in intravenous fluids has been discussed in Chapter 2. The main hazard is from Gram-negative bacilli growing to large numbers in the fluid, and every effort should be made to prevent this, by not leaving containers exposed for too long at room temperature after opening and keeping blood at 4°C. *Candida* spp. will also grow well in some fluids used for total parenteral nutrition. The principle is as usual to prevent the administration of large numbers of organism (either living or dead) to the patient.

Hepatitis B has been a worry in recent years particularly since the outbreaks in dialysis units in the early 1970s. Spread in hospital is mainly by needle pricks, although the virus can be isolated in secretions of carriers or infected patients. The risk of spread is greater from patients with acute infection when the virus concentration in the blood is high. Virus concentration may also be high in patients with renal failure. Infectivity also appears to be greater if the e-antigen can be detected in blood. Spread can occur from carriers of surface antigen ($HB_sAg$), but the risks are much less. The reduction in the incidence of hospital-acquired infection has been mainly due to increased care in dealing with infected patients and carriers, and screening of blood for transfusion. Improved hygienic techniques and care in handling blood and needles has considerably reduced the risks in surgery and in labour wards. Acquisition in laboratories is now rare. Airborne spread is not a major hazard although it is possible that infection could occur via the conjunctiva. Wearing of spectacles when operating on carriers is probably worthwhile, although the evidence for infection via this route suggests that in practice it is rare. Administration of vaccine to high risk groups should further reduce risks of infection.

The human immunodeficiency virus (HIV) is now causing considerable anxiety in health care workers, although there is little evidence of transfer to staff. It is transferred mainly by sexual intercourse, by blood transfusion or blood products. A small number of infections have occurred from injuries from needles used on infected patients. However, many needle stick injuries have occurred in health care workers throughout the world without transferring infection, whereas hepatitis B virus (HBV) has often been transferred by this route. It seems likely that the smaller number of HIV than HBV particles in the blood of infected patients considerably decreases the chance of infection. Several infections have also been reported from contamination of damaged skin by infected blood. HIV has been isolated from most body fluids, including saliva, but evidence available suggests spread by these routes is unlikely. The virus will survive for some days in exudate on surfaces, but indirect spread or airborne spread has not been reported. The virus is unstable and is more readily inactivated by chemical agents such as glutaraldehyde, hypochlorites, 70% ethanol, some detergents and heat than the hepatitis virus. The present routine tests available are for antibody which often appears several months after infection. This indicates that recently infected patients may not be detectable by HIV antibody tests. There is little evidence of surgeons or dentists acquiring an infection whilst operating on an infected patient, but one or two laboratory staff working with the virus have been infected. An infected mother may transfer infection to her baby during pregnancy, or during birth, but transfer by contact after birth is less likely. The virus has been isolated in breast milk, but spread by this route remains uncertain.

Creutzfeld-Jakob disease is characterized by progressive dementia and is transmitted by an agent called a 'slow virus'. It has been transmitted by organ transplant, contaminated brain electrodes and human growth hormone. The agent has not been grown in tissue culture and is believed to be a protein structure termed a 'prion', since no nucleic acid has been demonstrated. It is resistant to aldehydes, but can be inactivated by autoclaving at 132°C for 18 minutes and by strong hypochlorite solutions and sodium hydroxide.

# Chapter 4

# Outbreaks of infection and infectious diseases: investigation and action

The definition of an outbreak is often difficult, but for practical purposes in hospital it can be considered as two or more epidemiologically-related infections caused by an organism of the same type. The main problem is to identify common organisms as being similar in type as rapidly as possible (see Chapter 2). *E. coli* is a common cause of urinary tract infection and most infections due to sensitive strains are endogenous in origin. Several endogenous infections may occur in catheterized patients in a ward at the same time and a suitable rapid typing method is not usually available. If the strains are resistant to several antibiotics or one unusual antibiotic, such as gentamicin, cross-infection is a more likely explanation. Similarly, penicillin-resistant strains of *Staph. aureus* are commonly present in the nose of healthy carriers, and phage typing is necessary to determine whether strains are the same. Even then, certain types are common and could occur by chance in several patients in a ward at the same time. Several infections caused by methicillin- or gentamicin-resistant strains in a ward are suggestive of cross-infection and phage typing is less important. If the causative organisms are not commonly part of the normal flora, e.g. *Salmonella typhimurium,* two infections in one ward are likely to be an outbreak. This applies to a lesser extent to β-haemolytic streptococci which may be part of the normal flora, but typing of strains is preferable although it is unwise to await results before taking action. Epidemiological relationships are of importance. Wound infections caused by a similar type of *Staph. aureus* in three different wards may have a common origin in one operating theatre. However, if no connection can be found, the finding of the same strains in different wards is probably irrelevant. There are also situations in which one infection can be an indication for action. An infection occurring in a patient who has been in hospital for longer than the incubation period suggests a source in the hospital. A case of typhoid fever in a patient who has been in hospital for 4 weeks suggests a carrier should be sought.

The action taken varies with circumstances. Two minor staphylococcal infections caused by the same penicillin-resistant type may not be sufficient to take immediate action, but the situation should be carefully watched. If the two strains are gentamicin- and methicillin-resistant (or even if there is only one such strain) immediate action is indicated. Immediate action is sometimes needed if only one case e.g. diphtheria is identified in the hospital, but a single case of gastroenteritis may only require isolation and clinical surveillance of other patients. Screening of contacts is not usually required.

## Identification of the outbreak

The system of surveillance should detect potential outbreaks as quickly as possible[14]. Ward staff should be encouraged to send samples to the laboratory from all suspected infections. The laboratory staff should save certain reports for inspection by the Infection Control Nurse and should inform the microbiologist of any evidence suggesting a potential outbreak. Reports of the following should be inspected:

1. All wounds and bacteraemias.
2. All infections from the special care baby unit, intensive care, paediatric, other high risk areas and communicable diseases.
3. All *Pseudomonas aeruginosa*, Group A haemolytic streptococci, *Salmonella*, *Shigella*, enteropathogenic *E.coli* or rotavirus.
4. Highly resistant strains of *Staph. aureus*, or strains resistant to methicillin, fusidic acid or gentamicin, and highly-resistant Gram-negative bacilli (or resistant to gentamicin and other aminoglycosides).

The ward staff (medical and nursing) should also be encouraged to inform Infection Control Staff if infections are occurring in a ward; occasionally microbiological samples or reports are not immediately available, e.g. from a deep wound, or from a patient admitted with diarrhoea in the maternity department.

The decision to keep long-term records is difficult, but it is advisable to keep some (e.g. of 1–4 above) so that related infections occurring sporadically (e.g. one per week or one every few weeks in one ward) can be recognized. A 'Kardex' system with a page for each ward or unit is a convenient method. Computerized records are increasingly being used to identify a predetermined level of infection or to detect a specific organism. It is important that the information is regularly reviewed by the Infection Control Team.

## Assessment

On visiting the ward the Infection Control Nurse or Officer will determine the following:

1. Are the infections genuine or are the sites only colonized? Colonization may be an indication of a spreading organism, e.g. gentamicin-resistant *Staph. aureus* in several pressure sores, but may not be an indication for immediate action.
2. Are the infections hospital-acquired?
3. Are they likely to spread?
4. Is there any evidence of existing cross-infection?

A standard record or form will help to answer these questions. The following should be recorded if an outbreak of wound infection is suspected: ward or department; name, age, sex and hospital number of the patients involved; date of admission; date of onset; date and type of operation; whether the operation was drained; the time relationship of infection to ward dressings, operating theatre and surgeon; position of patient on operating list; organisms isolated and antibiotic sensitivity patterns; position of patient in ward; antibiotics given.

This information may be sufficient to make an immediate decision without further microbiology tests. For instance, if there are three infections due to different organisms, it is not an outbreak (although there may still be a need to investigate aseptic techniques). A deep infection in an undrained wound was probably acquired in the operating theatre. However, at this stage it may be necessary to decide on the necessity for further studies, e.g. nose swabs from staff, air-sampling or sampling of equipment. It may also be necessary to arrange for immediate isolation of certain patients, e.g. with a salmonella infection in a maternity unit. Comparison of infected and non-infected patients with similar underlying conditions (matched controls) may provide evidence of factors common to the infected patients, e.g. catheterization. The following should be considered when an outbreak occurs or a case of communicable disease is found in a ward:

1. Isolation of infected patients.
2. Consider the need for convening the Major Outbreaks Committee (see below).
3. Prevention of movement of staff to other wards.
4. Non-admission of new patients, unless immune.
5. Sending home of as many patients as possible.
6. Administration of immune serum to highly susceptible patients, e.g. leukaemics exposed to chicken-pox.
7. Treatment of contacts, e.g. erythromycin to close contacts with a case of diphtheria.
8. Informing administration (general, nursing and medical).
9. Introduction of new measures or improving existing procedures, e.g. alcohol disinfection of hands.
10. Closure of wards or introduction of cohort system in neonatal wards.
11. Sampling of contacts and environment.

The measures required will obviously have to be decided for each situation and occasionally some risks may be necessary and must be decided on probabilities. The closure of a ward and sampling faeces of all patients and staff when a single case of typhoid fever is recognized on a surgical ward is unnecessary. Typhoid rarely spreads from person to person, but it obviously can. Nevertheless, the risk is so small that it is not worth closing down an important surgical service.

It is necessary to keep everyone informed and all movements of patients should be decided with the co-operation of the relevant clinician who has the ultimate responsibility for his patients.

## Major outbreaks or infection problems requiring unusual measures[3]

These are difficult to define but usually consist of a large number of infections, e.g. *Salmonella, Legionella,* requiring additional facilities, materials or major staff changes. Examples include: closing of wards; opening a special isolation ward; more nursing, medical or domestic staff; more linen or CSSD materials; assistance from other hospitals, specialist laboratories or the Communicable Disease Surveillance Centre (CDSC). A single case of a particularly hazardous disease, e.g. Lassa fever or diphtheria, or an outbreak involving fatal cases or community involvement, may all require special action.

The Major Outbreaks Committee should be convened by a senior administrator and should consist of a senior member of the medical and nursing staff, Medical Officer of Environmental Health (if involving a notifiable disease or the community), the microbiologist and other Infection Control Staff. The Occupational Health physician or nurse, and infectious diseases physician, if available, should also be invited. The Infection Control Doctor or Chairman of the Infection Control Committee should co-ordinate the investigations and procedures (see also p. 3). In addition to the measures already mentioned, the following should be considered:

1. Nominating a person responsible for providing information to the media;
2. Obtaining outside assistance where necessary;
3. Notification to Regional Medical Officer, Department of Health, CDSC and other hospitals in the area.

Communication is particularly important within the hospital, and relevant information should be provided to relatives of infected patients as well as heads of departments, e.g. domestic, laundry, catering, CSSD and pharmacy.

# Outbreaks of surgical infection with *Staph. aureus*[15]

The following information is useful when considering an outbreak of staphylococcal wound infection:

1. Infection with antibiotic-sensitive organisms or strains resistant to penicillin only is likely to be endogenous in origin or acquired in the operating theatre. Multi-resistant strains are usually ward-acquired. However, strains may be acquired before operation, particularly if the length of stay is prolonged and then the infection appears to be endogenous although it was really hospital-acquired.
2. Sources are human, often with lesions, and are usually heavy dispersers. Healthy males are more likely to be dispersers and perineal carriers than females. Look for causes which might not be reported, e.g. pressure sores or fungal rashes.
3. The dry environment is not a major source or route of spread unless in close contact with the patient, e.g. bedclothes.
4. Undrained wounds seal in 1–2 days and infection acquired in the ward is then unlikely.

### Infections of theatre origin

Theatre infection is suspected if it is deep and in an undrained, clean, dry wound, or if an infection occurs before any ward dressing is carried out. Infection in drained wounds can originate either in the ward or in the theatre. Similar strains causing infections in different wards, but operated on by the same surgical team, are good evidence of theatre-acquired infection. Visit the theatre and find out which members of staff were present at the operations subsequently infected, and whether any of them has an infected lesion (or non-infected skin lesion, e.g. eczema). The source may be determined at this time with very little disturbance to staff or without much additional microbiology.
  If this fails:

1. Take nose swabs from all staff.
2. Sample the air during an operation performed by the suspect team, or sample the theatre floor with contact plates at the end of the operation.

If the organism is resistant to an antibiotic other than penicillin, it may usefully be incorporated into the culture media.

Sampling of the floors of the changing rooms may also be useful if the source is not identified by other means.

If no nasal carrier of the epidemic strain is found, but it is present in the environment, repeat nasal swabs and sample fingers of staff. If this fails, take perineal swabs and examine all staff for lesions. However, if noses and environment are both negative, continue close surveillance and repeat sampling if infections continue as some healthy carriers only disperse intermittently and for short periods.

### An example of an outbreak

A summary of four infections is shown in Table 5. An infection of a herniorrhaphy or a varicose vein operation is likely to be theatre-acquired and two different wards are involved. Infections occurred in Theatre 2 and the anaesthetist is a primary

**Table 5 Infections due to penicillin-resistant** *Staphylococcus aureus* **(phage type 52, 52A, 79)**

| Infected operation | Operating theatre | Ward | Surgeon | Anaesthetist |
|---|---|---|---|---|
| Hernia | 2 | 4 | Mr A | Dr B |
| Cholecystectomy | 2 | 1 | Mr C | Dr B |
| Hernia | 2 | 4 | Mr A | Dr B |
| Varicose veins | 2 | 1 | Mr A | Dr B |

suspect. If he is not a carrier of the epidemic strain, the staff and environment of Theatre 2 should be examined. Although a member of the scrubbed staff is the most likely source, others in the theatre at the time of the operation may be the source.

### Treatment of staphylococcal carrier

Dr B was found to be a nasal carrier of the epidemic strain. Dispersal tests were made as previously described and treatment was suggested as follows:

Daily baths with an antibacterial agent (chlorhexidine, povidone-iodine, triclosan or hexachlorophane detergent) for 1 week. Twice-weekly hair wash with one of the antibacterial detergents (cetrimide shampoo may be preferred). Nasal treatment with cream containing 1% chlorhexidine and 0.5% neomycin or other appropriate agent; cream should be applied to anterior nares four times a day for 1 week. Sample 2 days and 2 weeks after completing treatment (see p. 35).

### Problems of carriers

*How long should the person be off duty?*

If a superficial skin lesion is present the infected person should remain off duty until healed, or, if a groin rash, until free of *Staph. aureus*. If the person is a healthy nasal carrier and not a disperser he could return to duty after a few days treatment, but no one should continue as member of the scrubbed team until dispersal has ceased. Wherever possible a member of staff carrying a strain which has caused infection should not return to the operating theatre until that strain is removed. This decision may be difficult for a busy surgeon or anaesthetist and suppressive treatment for long periods should be considered, e.g. nose cream and antiseptic detergent for all washing and bathing for several months. If this fails a ventilated, bacteria-impermeable suit must be considered, although we have as yet no experience of this method.

*Failure of treatment*
Repeat courses of treatment should be tried, but in some individuals the strain still returns. Alternative nasal cream or antiseptic detergents may be tried. Clothing and bedding should be washed or dry-cleaned towards the end of a course of treatment and it may be necessary to investigate and treat other members of the family. Prolonged suppressive treatment as already described may be necessary. However, we have not yet failed to get a person back to duty either with the organism removed or suppressed, unless associated with chronic skin disease. In many instances, particularly if the colonized subject has a chronic skin disease, work elsewhere in the hospital may be possible.

*The staphylococcus is resistant to neomycin*
Chlorhexidine cream 1% alone or 1% hexachlorophane may be tried. Bacitracin cream may also be effective but is not so readily obtainable. Mupirocin 2% (pseudomonic acid) appears to be more effective than chlorhexidine preparations, particularly against methicillin-resistant staphylococci, but a few resistant strains have been reported. Gentamicin, fusidic acid, co-trimoxazole or vancomycin creams may all be effective, but are either expensive or are likely to cause the emergence of resistant strains. If any of these agents are used, treat for short periods only (not more than 2 weeks) and carefully follow up the treated person. A short systemic course of rifampicin and fusidic acid may be effective if other regimes fail and for throat carriers. However, there is always the risk of emergence of resistance to both agents, and careful monitoring is necessary.

**Outbreaks in the surgical ward**

Infected patients are the main sources (Figure 12).

*Investigation*
Nose swabs are taken from staff and patients, and swabs are taken from all wounds and lesions. Dispersers may be identified by exposing settle plates, by sampling floors or preferably by sweep or contact plates of bedding. If the epidemic strain is resistant to an antibiotic other than penicillin it can be incorporated into the culture media.

*Action*
Patients with infected lesions should be isolated or sent home and dispersers should be given a priority for isolation. Outbreaks often cease when the main disperser has been removed. Nasal carriers of the epidemic strain should be treated. This applies also to staff, although they are more often victims than causes. Other measures include the use of antiseptic detergents or 70% alcohol for handwashing or disinfection. Antiseptics, e.g. povidone-iodine, chlorhexidine, triclosan or hexachlorophane, should be added routinely to bath water. Infected patients or

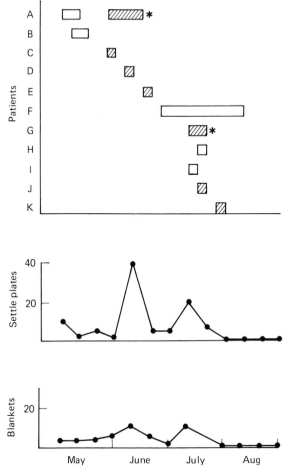

**Figure 12** Spread of *Staph. aureus* from dispersers A and G with increased air counts and blanket contamination; □, lesions; □, noses; *, heavy dispersers

carriers should bath and wash with an antiseptic detergent. If the epidemic continues nasal prophylaxis of all patients and staff should be considered. Wounds (infected or liable to infection) can often be sealed with an adhesive water vapour-permeable plastic sheet (e.g. Opsite), or covered with an antiseptic-impregnated dressing. Avoid use of topical antibiotics if possible.

### Staphylococcal outbreaks in a neonatal ward

Epidemic strains tend to be penicillin-resistant only and to colonize the nose, umbilicus and groins of babies. Spread is from baby to baby, usually via the hands of staff and not in the air. A member of staff or mother may introduce the strain initially into the nursery.

*Investigation*
Swabs should be taken from noses of nurses and babies and from the umbilicus of babies and any lesion. As in a surgical ward, dispersers may be detected by settle plates or sampling of bedding.

*Action*
Isolate infected babies with staphylococcal infection even if there is only one in the ward. If the strain is spreading cohort nursing should be introduced. Carriers should be treated with an antiseptic detergent and nose cream.

## Methicillin-resistant *Staphylococcus aureus* (MRSA)[16]

Methicillin-resistant strains are usually resistant to several additional antibiotics, e.g. tetracycline, erythromycin, neomycin, co-trimoxazole and often to gentamicin. Some show a particular propensity to spread and are termed epidemic strains (EMRSA), but there is no readily available laboratory test to detect them, and all MRSA must be treated with caution.

Investigation and control methods are similar to those already described. Isolation of the infected or colonized patient is particularly important in high risk units, e.g. intensive care, special care baby units, cardiothoroacic surgery units. Many strains spread without causing clinical infection, e.g. in a burns unit, and excessive efforts to eradicate them may not be in the interests of optimal patient care and would not be cost-effective. It is preferable to prevent strains from being brought into the unit. Detection, isolation and treatment of the first patient detected is the most important measure. The following should also be considered:

1. Nasal swabs alone will fail to detect many carriers. Swabs should be taken from nose, throat, perineum and all lesions including catheter sites, etc. Sampling of the bed sore area of bedridden patients, sputum, urine and faeces might also be considered, depending on the diagnosis. Screening of patients' fingers and bedding may reduce the need for initial multiple sampling.
2. Use mupirocin for treating nasal carriers and colonized sites. Patients should also have a daily bath with an antiseptic detergent. This should be extended to all patients during an outbreak. Staff, who are nasal carriers only, may return to work after 1–2 days treatment with mupirocin.
3. Mark patient's notes so that they can be detected early on re-admission or admission to another hospital. Strains may return after clear post-treatment screening samples. This may take several months.
4. Prevent movement of staff and patients as much as possible during an outbreak. Check whether agency staff are working in other hospitals with an MRSA problem.
5. Inform Infection Control Staff if patient is transferred to another hospital.

# Gram-negative bacilli

Most infections are endogenous and infected patients are the main sources in outbreaks, but common-source outbreaks can occur from equipment which comes into close contact with a susceptible site on the patient. Environmental sources are commonly fluids. Common organisms causing outbreaks are *Klebsiella/Enterobacter* spp. and *Ps. aeruginosa,* but can include *E. coli, Proteus* spp., other

*Pseudomonas* spp., *Serratia marcescens, Acinetobacter anitratus* and many other Gram-negative bacilli. Most of these, apart from *E. coli,* can survive well and grow in the moist environment of the ward. Infection has been reported from nebulizers, mechanical ventilators, disinfectant or antiseptic solutions, inadequately sterilized parenteral fluids or saline used at operation, hand creams, shaving brushes, transducers and monitoring equipment, endoscopes. Other possible sources are washing bowls, baths, nail-brushes, soap-dishes and containers, thermometer fluid, food-mixers, mattresses, urine bottles and bedpans.

The history of the patient may indicate a common source. In an outbreak of *Ps. aeruginosa* in a neurosurgical unit, the organism was only found on the scalp after shaving. Although *Ps. aeruginosa* was widely distributed in the environment, none was the epidemic strain, apart from one strain in a shaving brush (Figure 13) which was considered to be the common source.

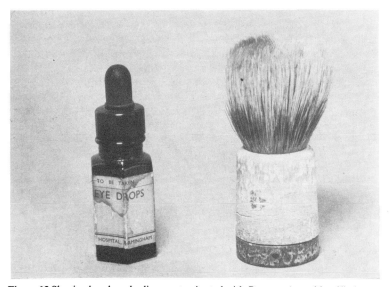

**Figure 13** Shaving brush and saline contaminated with *Ps. aeruginosa* identified as sources of outbreaks

**Table 6 Phage patterns of *Ps. aeruginosa* isolated from an eye hospital during an outbreak of infection**

| Site of isolation | Phage pattern |
| --- | --- |
| Bath and sink (bathroom) | 7/31/73 |
| Floor, sink, cloth (sluice room) | 7/31/73/109/119X |
| Floor and sink (ward) | 7/21/68/119X |
| Urine bottles + mop and bucket (1) | 7/31/73 |
| + mop and bucket (2) | 109/119X |
| Saline used to irrigate eyes | 7/24/68/1214 |
| Eye infections | 7/24/68/1214 |

Phage patterns from environment, apart from saline, differ from those causing infection

A similar study in an eye hospital, in which a number of patients lost their sight, showed that the strain was present in saline used to moisten the eye at operation. Phage typing results are shown in Table 6.

In neonatal units, a source in the labour ward should be sought if infections are occurring within a few days of birth. Suction equipment is always a possibility. Other moist areas, such as baths, soaps, etc. should be examined.

It is important that infections arising from contaminated intravenous fluids are identified rapidly. The contents of the container should be sampled as soon as possible and the batch number referred to the pharmacy so that suspect bottles can be withdrawn from circulation. Unusual organisms, e.g. *Erwinia,* in a blood culture should alert Infection Control Staff to the possibility and careful surveillance is important, preferably on a national scale.

## Investigation

Information is collected on the patients with infection and should include time of indwelling catheterization, mechanical respiratory ventilation, intravenous cannu-lation, antibiotic therapy, as well as the usual data on age, length of stay, diagnosis, treatment with steroids, etc. Samples should be collected from all patients where appropriate, e.g. sputa, catheter specimens of urine, wounds, bed sores and other lesions. The indications may be of patient-to-patient cross-infection. It may then be worthwhile looking at ward techniques, in particular catheter care and respiratory suction. In some instances, a common source may seem likely, and sampling of the relevant item of equipment or fluid is necessary. If the source is still unknown, general environmental sampling should be undertaken. This may bring to light deficiencies not previously recognized, e.g. inadequate disinfection of urine bottles, a bedpan washer/disinfector not working, failure to change tubing attached to a ventilator, topping-up of disinfectant solutions. The hands of the staff should also be sampled. This will demonstrate the importance of handwashing. Typing of strains may be necessary to differentiate between the epidemic strain and others. It must also be realized that equipment may be contaminated from the infected patients and not vice versa; this applies particularly to organisms in mops and sinks[8].

## Action

On completion of the epidemiological investigation it should be possible to prevent the spread of the organism by good aseptic techniques and adequate disinfection. An antiseptic detergent or alcoholic solution could be introduced for hand disinfection. If one patient is an obvious source, isolation in a single room may be worthwhile although the air is not a major route of spread (see Chapter 5).

# Legionnaires' disease[17]

Spread is usually in aerosols from air conditioning systems. Infection may also occur from nebulizers or whirlpools, showers or hot water supplies. Person-to-person spread does not occur. The elderly, particularly with pre-existing respiratory disease, or immunosuppressed patients are particularly susceptible. Early detection is important and this is usually based on clinical suspicion.

Although the organisms can sometimes be detected in sputum or bronchial washings, diagnosis is often only possible with an antibody test carried out at a later stage of the illness. Isolation of the patient is unnecessary. If the patient has been in hospital for 10 days or more, it is likely to be hospital-acquired. Look for other possible cases, but if none are found further investigation is not necessary. Two or more related cases require investigation. Samples of water (5 litres) should be collected from all possible sources, e.g. water tanks, hot and cold supplies, showers and cooling towers before any control measures are implemented.

Measures include raising the temperature of hot water supplies and additional chlorination. Neither method is entirely satisfactory; temperatures over 55°C are likely to scald elderly people and higher than usual chlorine levels may cause corrosion in the systems. In the event of a major outbreak, convene the Major Outbreaks Committee and consider asking for assistance from local PHLS laboratories or the Communicable Disease Surveillance Centre.

## Intestinal infection (*Salmonella, Shigella,* enteropathogenic *E.coli*)

If there is evidence of cross-infection with an intestinal pathogen involving two patients or more, samples of faeces should be collected from all patients and staff with diarrhoea *after* discussion with infection control staff. A history should be taken from infected patients and should include food and drugs taken over the past 48 hours. The infected patients should be isolated if possible in a single room with excretion precautions, and always if in a neonatal ward. If isolation is not possible, excretion precautions should still be introduced in the ward, e.g. handwashing after handling patient or surroundings, and care in disposal of faeces, handling bedpans and soiled linen. It may also be possible to nurse all infected patients together in one ward. If the outbreak is long and likely to require additional staff or facilities, the Major Outbreaks Committee should be convened (see p. 30)

It may be advisable to close the ward to new admissions and not to transfer staff to other wards. Neonatal wards should always be closed to new admissions if a known pathogen has spread. If an organism is identified, e.g. *Salmonella* or *Shigella,* faeces should be taken from all patients and sampling of staff should be considered; discuss this with the microbiologist before carrying out any mass sampling. The ward can be reopened when diarrhoea has ceased, but preferably when the pathogen can no longer be isolated from faeces. In general, two negative specimens from known cases should be sufficient. However, it may be necessary in some instances to reopen the ward whilst carriers still remain, although they should preferably be isolated.

If it seems likely that food is incriminated, e.g. all cases have eaten the same food, but not matched controls, and infection occurs throughout the hospital at the same time, catering practices and staff require investigation (Chapter 14). Often there will be no evidence of food-borne infection and no pathogen will be isolated. In this case carry out excretion precautions until symptoms cease; avoid admitting new patients, if possible. Check the disinfection of crockery and cutlery.

These infections are often viral in paediatric or geriatric departments and rotavirus may be detected in the faeces but often a diagnosis is not made. Nevertheless the measures outlined should still be applied.

## Infectious diseases of childhood

These commonly occur in paediatric wards and a succession of cases can occur in a ward over many months if adequate action is not taken. The common infections, chicken-pox, measles, rubella, mumps, can usually be readily identified and outbreaks are easily recognized by clinical means. The infected child should be isolated or sent home. If more than one, they can be nursed together in one ward. Susceptible children who may be harmed by the infection, e.g. leukaemics, those on steroids or other immunosuppressive drugs or with chronic diseases of the chest, heart or kidneys, should be given gammaglobulin.

A particular problem is that of susceptible staff. If it is decided to keep the ward open to all admissions, an infected member of staff could be responsible for further cases, even if the original case was isolated before spread had occurred to other patients. It is preferable to employ staff who have had the disease, or have been immunized, e.g. against measles and rubella, but this is not always known. Female staff not immune to rubella should not work on paediatric, isolation or maternity wards. A major problem is in an isolation ward which includes infected and susceptible patients. Patients with chicken-pox or measles should not be nursed by staff who are also attending immunosuppressed patients unless there is reasonably certain evidence of previous infection or immunity.

It is unnecessary to clean or disinfect wards after occupation by patients with childhood diseases as infection from the environment does not occur.

When to close wards is a difficult problem and is discussed below.

## Tuberculosis

It is usual to isolate patients with open pulmonary tuberculosis for the first few weeks of treatment. The period of isolation is uncertain, but from animal experiments and clinical experience the risk of spread after 2 weeks' effective treatment should be small and most of the organisms in the sputum should be non-viable. Exceptions will occur where the response is slow or the organisms are resistant to the antibiotics used, so that it is necessary to be careful in making hard and fast rules on length of time of isolation. A longer period of isolation (e.g. 4 weeks) should be carried out on paediatric wards.

Protecting the staff from acquiring respiratory infections by wearing masks is another uncertainty. It is unlikely that conventional masks will provide adequate protection, but may be advisable when dealing with severe disease. It may be more logical for the patient to wear the mask particularly when receiving close attention. The risks to staff immunized or naturally immune to tuberculosis appear to be small.

If a case of open pulmonary tuberculosis is found in a general ward, the immunity of the staff should be checked with the Occupational Health Department. Staff with a previously positive Mantoux or Heaf test or with evidence of successful BCG immunization require no further tests, but all contacts should be asked to report if they develop a chronic cough over the next 6 months.

Patient contacts are more difficult as many may have gone home. The general practitioners of known close contacts should be informed and patients told to visit them if symptoms occur. Spread from one patient to another is infrequent and it is of doubtful value following up large numbers of patients, most of whom have had limited or no close contact with the patient. However, the risk of spread is greater on paediatric wards and follow-up of contacts is more important.

# Hepatitis B (HBV) and human immune deficiency virus (HIV) infections[18]

Although outbreaks of HBV infection in hospitals are rare and spread of HIV infection is unlikely to be a major problem (see p. 26), measures are necessary to protect staff and patients.

### General precautions

Since unknown hepatitis carriers or HIV antibody-positive patients may be admitted with another diagnosis, some general measures are recommended:

1. Lesions on hands should be covered with a waterproof dressing. If not possible, e.g. if hands are chapped or because of dermatitis, gloves should be worn if contact with blood or secretions is likely. In units or hospitals where the incidence of HIV positive patients is likely to be high, gloves should be worn for all procedures involving contact with blood or secretions. In the USA, gloves are recommended for all blood contact. This is probably unnecessary in hospitals where HIV positive patients are rare, but this recommendation is increasingly being introduced into control of infection policies.
2. If skin or conjunctiva is accidentally contaminated with blood, wash immediately and thoroughly.
3. Needles should generally not be recapped. Replacing a needle into its protective sheath held in the opposing hand increases the risk of needle stick injury to the person doing it and needles should normally be discarded into an approved sharps box. If recapping is necessary a safe technique must be used, e.g. the needle holder can either be stood upright on the bench held in a suitable holder, e.g. plasticine, or held in a device which protects the hand.
4. If the skin is punctured with a needle or other sharp instrument, encourage bleeding, wash thoroughly and report to supervisor. Hepatitis B immunoglobulin may be required. Hepatitis B vaccine should be offered to all high risk groups.
5. Blood spillage should be cleaned up rapidly using gloves (see Chapter 10).

### Known carriers or infected patients

The above precautions are applicable, but gloves should always be worn taking blood if contact with blood is likely. A plastic apron to protect clothing is recommended.

Goggles or spectacles are advised for surgical teams during operations or obstetric staff for deliveries, although aerosol spread is unlikely and there is little evidence of infection via the conjunctiva available for HBV and none for HIV.

Permission should be given by the patient before blood is tested for HIV antibody and counselling should be provided on possible consequences of a positive test. An exception may be acceptable if the test is required for the differential diagnosis in an ill patient or a low risk patient. The clinician in charge of the patient should make this decision. Blood must be taken by experienced staff, the laboratory must be informed and the samples labelled 'Biohazard', but every effort should be made to ensure confidentiality.

Used equipment and linen (particularly if blood-stained) should also be labelled 'Biohazard' and treated accordingly (see p. 105). Blood spillage should be cleaned up with hypochlorite solution or powder (see p. 91).

Isolation is unnecessary, unless for other purposes, e.g. severe diarrhoea or tuberculosis in AIDS patients. Most infections in AIDS patients, e.g. *Pneumocystis carinii* or viral pneumonia, are not a hazard to staff.

# Other infectious diseases

Severe infections or potentially dangerous infections, such as diphtheria, are now rare and a case tends to cause an excessive response in the staff unless everyone is informed of the risks. All departments likely to be involved such as the laundry, CSSD and domestic departments should be informed. Little action is required in the hospital other than prophylactic treatment of close contacts where appropriate, e.g. erythromycin for diphtheria, rifampicin for meningococcal meningitis (not usually necessary for hospital staff). The MOEH should always be informed as investigations in families or schools may be necessary, and he has legal responsibilities for dealing with these infections.

# Lassa fever and other viral haemorrhagic diseases[19]

Patients with these infections will usually be nursed in high security units and will not be discussed further. However, the patients may be initially admitted to a casualty department or possibly to a ward in a general hospital. The following measures are therefore suggested:

### Patient admitted to a casualty department

1. A patient, particularly if a member of a hospital staff, presenting with symptoms of viral haemorrhagic fever during a 3-week period after arrival from a rural area of West Africa should be transferred to a designated isolation room in the department. The patient should not be allowed to leave this room until agreed by the Infection Control Officer.
2. The casualty officer or clinician diagnosing the infection should inform the duty consultant physician and the Infection Control Officer who will inform an infectious diseases consultant if necessary.
3. On instructions from the Infection Control Officer the senior nurse on duty will close the department to all further admissions and allow no patients or staff to leave. He/she will also inform the Infection Control Nurse, senior nursing officer on duty and the duty administrator.
4. Before transferring to the isolation room, remove all unnecessary equipment and the box containing protective clothing from the room. A notice 'Strict isolation – no not enter' should be placed on the door. One person only should accompany the patient into the room (a doctor or nurse who has already had close contact with the patient). This person should dress in a long-sleeved

disposable gown, cap, filter-type mask and overshoes. These articles are provided in a special box contained in the isolation room. Urine and faeces should be collected in a disposable pan or urinal and sealed in a plastic bag.

If the infectious diseases consultant thinks a diagnosis of viral haemorrhagic fever is likely he will arrange for the transfer of the patient to a special unit and inform the Medical Officer of Environmental Health (MOEH).

Then:

1. The casualty sister, Infection Control Nurse and administrator will collect names and addresses of all contacts and allow them to leave on agreement with the MOEH. The Infection Control Nurse and Occupational Health Nurse will be responsible for tracing other hospital contacts and the MOEH for persons outside the hospital.
2. After the patient is removed to the ambulance, the person attending the patient will remove protective clothing and seal in plastic bag, and leave the room. The door should be sealed with tape until the MOEH has made arrangements for decontamination of the room and its contents and disposal of potentially infected materials.
3. The administrator will call a meeting of the Major Outbreaks Committee (MOEH, Infection Control Officer and Nurse, consultant physician, senior nurse and Occupational Health Nurse or Physician, see p. 30).

### Patient in a ward

1. The doctor in charge will inform the consultant physician and the Infection Control Officer who will inform an infectious diseases consultant if necessary.
2. Transfer the patient to a side room.
3. The senior nurse in the ward will inform the Infection Control Nurse (who will bring the box containing protective clothing) and the senior nursing officer on duty in the hospital.
4. A notice 'Strict isolation – do not enter' is placed on the door. One doctor or nurse should accompany the patient into the ward and should dress in the protective clothing.
5. Do not take any laboratory specimens until agreed by the infectious diseases consultant.

If the infectious diseases consultant thinks the suspected infection is likely he will arrange for transport to the special unit and inform the MOEH. The infection control and occupational health nurses will collect names of contacts, not forgetting laboratory staff who may have handled specimens, as well as radiology or physiotherapy staff where relevant. The admission of a suspected patient to a general hospital should be avoided if possible. General practitioners should request a visit by the infectious diseases consultant at the patient's home. The Major Outbreaks Committee will be called and decontamination procedures decided, as well as any quarantine arrangements.

## Closure of wards

This is a major step which reduces the efficiency of the hospital and should be avoided if possible. It should be unnecessary for staphylococcal or Gram-negative infections, since spread can usually be controlled by isolation of selected patients, good techniques and special control measures. A heavy staphylococcal disperser of an epidemic strain should be removed from the ward and nursed in a side ward (possibly associated with a medical ward) which should be available somewhere in the hospital even if in short supply. Neonatal wards should be closed if there is evidence of spread, but cohort nursing is often possible. Every general hospital should have an isolation unit, particularly if side rooms are inadequate. Spread of MRSA may be difficult to control and may require closure of wards, particularly surgical or intensive care.

Infectious diseases in paediatric wards present one of the more important problems. If a single case of chicken-pox or measles occurs, should the ward be closed to non-immune admissions? Spread may not occur, but on the other hand the epidemic may continue for months. An alternative may be to send home contacts in the early stages of the incubation period and isolate long-stay non-immune contacts. If a disease is common in the community and cases are continually being admitted, closure may not be worthwhile.

# Chapter 5

# Factors associated with wound, chest and urinary tract infection and general measures for prevention

## Surgical wounds[20-22]

Infection may he acquired during the operation or postoperatively in the ward (see also Chapters 3 and 4). During the operation it may he acquired from the skin, respiratory or gastrointestinal tract of the patient, or from the skin or upper respiratory tract of the operating room staff, either by contact or through the air. Infection may also be acquired from contaminated equipment. Airborne spread is likely to be due to *Staph. aureus,* or possibly *Staph. epidermidis* in implant surgery[23]. Small numbers of *Staph. aureus* are usually present in the air of a normally ventilated theatre. The numbers falling into a wound during an operation are likely to be small, but a single skin scale may be carrying up to 100 or more individual cocci. The chances of a large enough inoculum reaching the wound and causing an infection are increased by the following:

### Factors influencing infection

1. A long incision and a long operating time, as in cardiothoracic surgery.
2. A heavy disperser of *Staph. aureus* in the theatre, especially if a member of the operating team.
3. Many peopie in the theatre or considerable activity during the operation.
4. The technique of the surgeon is inadequate and the wound edges are too tightly or loosely opposed; this may be difficult to avoid in obese patients. A haematoma may occur in the wound.
5. The organisms land on an ischaemic area or an artificial implant.
6. The wound is drained, particularly if drainage is not closed.
7. The patient is particularly susceptible, e.g. very young, old, or has a pre-existing disease – cardiac, respiratory, diabetes, a malignant growth, or is suffering from malnutrition, obesity or is immunosuppressed.
8. The skin of the patient is colonized with a potential pathogen or there is an area of superficial sepsis on another site of the body.

The hands of the surgeon or skin of the operation site are rarely colonized with *Staph. aureus,* and Gram-negative bacilli are usually removed by simple washing processes. The importance of glove punctures is over-emphasized in general surgery. Although the host defences and surgical technique are the main factors, it must be ensured that:

1. The hands of the surgeon and the skin of the operation site are disinfected and no one with superficial sepsis is in the theatre.
2. The ventilation system is working efficiently.
3. Instruments, operation gowns, drapes, etc. are sterile (rarely a problem).

Good surveillance will detect outbreaks and enable dispersers to be detected on subsequent investigation.

Short-term antibiotic prophylaxis may be of value in contaminated or high risk surgery, cardiac and joint prostheses, and should be individually assessed.

### Ward-acquired infection

The site of acquisition of infection (i.e. ward or theatre) varies with different sites of operation and in different wards or hospitals. Clean and undrained wounds seal rapidly in 1–2 days and are unlikely to be infected in the ward. It would seem that most infections are acquired in the operating theatre, but several ward factors are possibly relevant.

There is evidence of increasing ward infection rates with increased length of preoperative stay, with shaving on the day before operation or earlier and in drained wounds. It is also possible that infection would be reduced if shaving was avoided. Preoperative bathing with an antiseptic may reduce wound infection in certain types of surgery (e.g. vascular) but a single antiseptic bath as a routine is unlikely to have any effect[24]. Two or more antiseptic baths may be of value but the evidence is controversial[25, 26]. Infection is also more likely in overcrowded large wards, but it is possible that some of these factors are now less important since most of this information was obtained when staphylococcal cross-infection in the ward was a common cause of wound infection. However, the return of the MRSA has been associated with an increase in cross-infection in some hospitals.

Nevertheless, it seems rational to consider the following measures whenever possible:

1. Admit the patient to hospital as close to the time of operation as possible.
2. Shaving is usually unnecessary but excessive hair may be removed by clipping or depilation. If shaving is carried out it should be done on the day of operation[27].
3. Do not take ward bedding into the theatre.

   After operation:

4. Seal the wound thoroughly for 1–2 days.
5. Use closed drainage system (if a drain is required).
6. Discharge the patient as soon as possible.

The likelihood of a wound becoming infected during a dressing change is slight, particularly if closed. However, there is some evidence that infections of high risk wounds (e.g. cardiovascular) can occur in the recovery room and high aseptic standards are required.

Dressings should not be required on the wound after 48 hours. If removed at this time or before, the conflict between nursing staff requiring good aseptic techniques and surgeons lifting dressings with their hands will not occur. A simplified technique for changing dressings could be developed (see Chapter 6). However, patients with wounds infected or colonized with potentially epidemic strains of *Staph. aureus* should be isolated.

## Chest infection

Hospital-acquired or associated chest infection is often endogenous, occurring in patients with existing respiratory disease. Postoperative chest infection is commonly caused by *Haemophilus influenzae* or *Strep. pneumoniae*. Instrumentation is an important predisposing factor, e.g. endotracheal tubes and tracheostomies tend to bypass the normal respiratory defence system. Predisposing factors are old age, coma, excessive smoking, obesity, burns or major injury. The organisms associated with instrumentation or mechanical ventilation are mainly Gram-negative bacilli, such as *Klebsiella* spp. or *Ps. aeruginosa*. Colonization of the throat or tracheostomy wound with these organisms is common and usually does not harm the patient. However, an infection, indicated by purulent sputum, pyrexia and radiological changes, requires chemotherapy.

Gram-negative bacilli may be acquired from infected or colonized patients on the hands of staff, from food or from contaminated equipment. Endogenous infection is not readily prevented by the usual cross-infection measures but may be prevented to some extent by physiotherapy (see p. 123).

The essentials of prevention of Gram-negative infection are: effective handwashing between patients, decontamination of equipment – ventilators (change tubing every 48 hours[28]), humidifiers, washing bowls, shaving brushes, food-mixers, and other items likely to come into close contact with the patient. Antibiotics should be used with care; ampicillin tends to select *Klebsiella,* and spread to other patients is a particular hazard in strains highly resistant to antibiotics. Stopping antibiotics and isolation of patients with resistant strains are important steps in controlling an epidemic.

## Urinary tract infection[29] (see also Chapter 6)

Although infection can occur via the bloodstream, the commonest route is along the urethra. Infection without instrumentation is commoner in the female owing to the short urethra. However, hospital-acquired urinary tract infection usually occurs after instrumentation. The organisms are usually of faecal origin and may be found on the perineum or in the anterior urethra. Coagulase-negative staphylococci or micrococci are normally found in the anterior urethra and are a common cause of infection immediately after catheterization. Early infections are usually endogenous, but cross-infection occurs later in patients with an indwelling catheter. The use of a closed-drainage system considerably reduces the incidence of urinary tract infection in patients with indwelling catheters (Table 7), but infection still frequently occurs after about 7 or more days.

**Table 7 Urinary tract infections in females with indwelling catheters[30]**

| Treatment | Infection rate during drainage |
|---|---|
| Open drainage | 29/34(85%) |
| Closed drainage | 18/47(38%) |
| Closed drainage (with anchored catheter) | 5/29 (17%) |

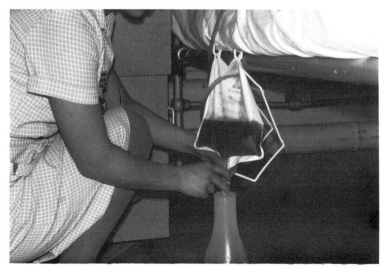

**Figure 14** Contamination of hands when emptying urine bag

Organisms may reach the bladder along the outside of the catheter or along the lumen, possibly in an air bubble. They may gain access to the closed drainage system if the catheter is disconnected from the system or from the tap used to empty the bag (Figure 14).

It is not possible to define the main route of infection. In late infection spread along the outside of the catheter is likely, but attempts to prevent this by applications of topical antibiotics or disinfectants to the catheter–meatal junction have not been successful. Anchoring the catheter in females has achieved some success, as movement of the catheter in the short female urethra is a likely way of introducing infection. However, if the urethra is colonized, treatment of the catheter–meatal junction is unlikely to have much influence. Retrograde spread from the bag or container along the lumen of the catheter is probably also important. Unfortunately, the non-return valve in the drainage bag is rarely effective. Tests in the laboratory in which a contaminated bag was tipped at intervals showed that growth reached the 'patient' end of the catheter in 2–3 days. Patients often swing or sit on drainage bags. How do the organisms get into the bag? A few may be excreted in normal urine and grow in the drainage bag. Retrograde spread of large numbers of the patient's own organisms may cause a bladder infection. Although disinfectant in the bag may be considered useful, trials have not usually confirmed a preventative effect. Cross-infection from other patients is more important and is likely to occur via the hands of staff, contaminating the catheter–meatal junction, disconnecting the catheter, or contaminating the tap when emptying the drainage bag.

The fingers of the nurse are often contaminated with large numbers of organisms when emptying the bag and handling the container in which the bag is emptied. Unless the hands are thoroughly washed (or gloves are worn) between patients and a clean container is used, organisms are readily transferred to the next patient. The catheter–meatal junction may be contaminated when the patients use a toilet, commode or bedpan or during bathing. The hands of patients with a urinary infection are often heavily contaminated and may transfer infection to the hands of others who may subsequently contaminate their own catheter–meatal junction or perineum. Some organisms seem likely to spread, e.g. antibiotic-resistant *Klebsiella*. Cross-infection tends to occur if antibiotics are widely used in a unit and there are a number of patients with indwelling catheters, particularly if they are in adjacent beds or sit together during the day.

Infection may be acquired in non-catheterized patients, although the route of spread is uncertain. Contamination of urine bottles, bedpans and urine-testing equipment have all been associated with outbreaks. Contamination of tanks of disinfectant with Gram-negative bacilli have been reported on occasions.

It has been suggested that intermittent catheterization is less likely to be followed by infection than indwelling catheterization, but the evidence is doubtful. However, there is some evidence that infection after suprapubic catheterization is less than with an indwelling catheter.

### General measures

Avoid catheterization if possible, particularly in incontinent patients. Remove the catheter as soon as possible (within 5 days). Collect urine specimens with a syringe by inserting the needle through a sleeve in the tubing of the drainage set. Disinfect urinals and bedpans preferably by heat in urology wards, and wash hands between emptying bags (disinfection of hands with 70% alcohol is rapid and effective). It is also preferable to wear gloves. Containers in which drainage bags are emptied should be clean and dry (preferably disinfected by heat). Restriction in the use of broad-spectrum antibiotics (antibiotics are relatively ineffective in the presence of an indwelling catheter), but a short prophylactic course to cover the instrumentation period may prevent bacteraemia and reduce infection in the first few days of continuous catheterization, particularly if the patient already has a urinary tract infection.

### During an outbreak (see also Chapter 4)

In addition to the above measures, separation of patients with indwelling catheters in the ward is advisable. Isolate patients with highly resistant strains. Introduce alcoholic disinfection of hands after handling infected patients or their immediate environment.

# Chapter 6

# Nursing aspects of prevention of infection: aseptic and hygienic techniques

## Relating infection control to nursing practice

Infection control practices need to be integrated into the nursing procedures of each hospital. This means that problems of infection control should be identified in each clinical area and included in the care plans for individual patients. The equipment and procedures used will vary from one hospital to another and will need to be critically assessed to ensure that infection risk has been minimized. Methods should be sufficiently flexible to adapt to patient needs without increasing that risk. Although infections are classified as wound, urinary tract, enteric infections, etc., it is important to remember that it is an individual who becomes infected and that the infection is likely to cause emotional as well as physical distress. Unnecessary measures can exaggerate the severity of the problem in the minds of the patients, their families and friends. Wherever practical, the reason for the measures taken should be explained in a language appropriate to the individual. Measures applied to an infected patient are often taken to protect other more vulnerable patients, and the risk to families and visitors may be very low. Explaining this can be reassuring to the infected patient and relatives.

Each patient should be seen as part of the nursing environment interacting in a specific way with that environment and the other patients. The presence of a patient may increase infection risk to others, or other patients may increase the risk to him. The distribution of patients within the ward can be important even where isolation is not required.

The complexity of this interaction is apparent when considering individual patients. An elderly lady recovering from a hip prosthesis operation is likely to be vulnerable to a different range of organisms from those infecting a patient following colonic surgery. Her age may make her more vulnerable than a much younger person having the same operation. Inadequate nursing care may lead to pressure sores, which may then become a potential source of infection to other patients. Previous antibiotic treatment for chronic bronchitis may have caused colonization of carriage sites with antibiotic-resistant organisms which could increase infection risk both to the patient and others in contact with her. Catheterization may become necessary and result in urinary tract infection. About one-third of all hospital-acquired infections are of the urinary tract, most of which are associated with catheterization. Nursing care must be planned with an awareness of the measures that increase infection risk and the use of these techniques balanced against the possible benefits. The care plan for this patient could include a high fluid intake and bladder training so that catheterization can be avoided, frequent mouth toilet to prevent oral thrush, frequent turning and attention to pressure areas to prevent bed sores, early mobilization to prevent chest infection. Infection control measures need to be related to the requirements of each individual patient. Appropriate measures will not be the same for each patient, and even when the same measure is adopted for several patients, the priority given to that measure may be different. It is a waste of valuable resources to apply unnecessary infection control measures, but failure to apply necessary ones may indicate a lack of professional judgement.

**Risk assessment**

It should therefore be part of the nursing process to assess the infection risk for each individual patient. It is too easy to neglect infection amongst the many other priorities. A decision that 'it is not really necessary to wash the hands on this occasion' or 'the dressing does not really need changing quite as often as prescribed' is often made. Such decisions on priorities are required, but it is important to be aware that decisions on acceptable risks are being made on the patients' behalf and not for the convenience of staff; the patient, not the nurse, becomes infected if the decision is wrong.

Risk assessment is a measure of the probability of a person becoming infected. The immunological competence of the patient, the medical condition, the procedures which can reasonably be expected to be carried out during the hospital stay, need to be taken into consideration. The environment in which those procedures will be carried out and other individuals who will share the environment with the patient are also relevant to risk.

Most hospital infections occur because the patient was exposed to micro-organisms when particularly vulnerable. The organisms involved are rarely unusual in virulence or other properties, but are able to reach a normally inaccessible susceptible site on the patient because of a particular procedure. Approximately 60% of hospital-acquired infections are caused by common Gram-negative bacteria that are either normal inhabitants of the gut or can be found in almost any used or static fluid, i.e. opportunistic pathogens. Other more specific human infections, e.g. salmonellosis or childhood infectious diseases, may be acquired in hospital because the chance of contact is increased, often at a time when the ability to resist infection is decreased. This decrease may be due to disease, e.g. leukaemia, HIV infection or to the use of drugs which reduce immunological competence. It is because infection risk is associated with the reaction of the individual to his environment that advice may sometimes appear inconsistent; apparently irrelevant questions may be asked by infection control specialists in an attempt to establish which set of interactions are relevant on any specific occasion.

Risks will also vary in relative importance, and priorities will depend on the number of people likely to be infected, the severity of the resulting infection and how readily the infection responds to treatment. A hospital chef with *Salmonella* infection could infect hundreds, if not thousands, of patients if catering practice is poor. A single case of diphtheria may require immediate action since the consequence of spread could be severe. The nurse with an uncovered infected finger could cause infections in many of the wounds of patients who had been dressed by her over the next few days. Accidently touching a sterile dressing during a dressing procedure could infect the patient but the probability is not high.

Transferring *Staph. aureus* to cutlery while handing it to a patient could infect him, but the probability is again so remote that it can usually be ignored. Resources devoted to preventing infection should be related to the degree of risk involved.

Infection control may not be the major factor to be considered when carrying out a procedure and where action is required the wider implications must also be considered. It is normally advised that the same nurse should not attend an infectious patient and a heavily immunosuppressed patient on the same shift. This instruction may, however, be justifiably overridden in a sufficiently severe medical emergency, e.g. a patient choking by swallowing his tongue. In such a circumstance it might be unwise to spend time washing the hands before taking action.

### Seeking advice

The Infection Control Nurse should be a readily available source of advice, and it is a major part of her role to interpret policies; if in doubt – ask. Do not, however, be surprised if you are then asked questions; the question of which disinfectant to use may be inappropriate for a situation in which cleaning may be sufficient or sterilization may be necessary. Where recommendations are made to cope with new problems, feedback is essential. Did it work and is it likely to occur sufficiently often to include in procedure manuals or codes of practice?

## Measures to prevent infection

Infection control procedures may be generalized guidelines or policy decisions which may be either non-clinical, e.g. catering, domestic practice, laundering, waste disposal, etc., or clinical, e.g. policies for isolation of patients, use of antibiotics, etc., or involving both clinical and non-clinical areas, e.g. disinfectant policies. There may also be detailed guidance for specific procedures, e.g. catheterization. Policies should be sufficiently comprehensive to cover most eventualities, easily followed and unambiguous. They should also be well publicised and readily available. Some flexibility to allow policies to be adapted for the requirements of individual patient care is required. Nurses should make themselves aware of existing policies when changing from one ward to another or from one hospital to another.

### Handwashing in wards

Handwashing or disinfection is the most important technique in the prevention of cross-infection. However, apart from the studies of Semmelweiss and one or two studies in neonatal nurseries, there is little statistical evidence to confirm this statement. Many investigations have demonstrated the control of an outbreak by improving handwashing techniques, but this has usually been in association with other measures. Nevertheless, it is rational to consider that the hands of staff represent one of the main routes of spread. The problems to be considered are agents and techniques used and indications for handwashing.

Laboratory studies have demonstrated that washing with soap and water will remove or kill approximately 99% ($10^2$), antiseptic detergents approximately $10^2$–$10^3$) and 60–70% alcohol $10^3$–$10^4$ of transient organisms from the hands (Table 8)[31]. Although statistically significant differences between washing with soap and a

**Table 8 Hygienic hand disinfection (*E.coli* applied to finger tips)**

| Preparations | No. of tests | Mean log reduction |
|---|---|---|
| 70% Isopropanol | 9 | 3.3 |
| 70% Ethanol | 5 | 2.7 |
| 4% Chlorhexidine detergent | 2 | 2.9 |
| 7.5% Povidone-iodine | 4 | 2.5 |
| 2% Triclosan detergent | 2 | 2.3 |
| Unmedicated soap | 13 | 2.1 |

disinfectant may be obtained, the clinical relevance of a statistical difference (log 0.5–1.0) is much less certain.

Interpretation of laboratory results is difficult and the results should be assessed as indications of the order of effectiveness rather than an indication of specific reductions of organisms likely to be obtained under practical circumstances. To determine a clinically significant difference between a soap and water wash and an antiseptic wash it would require a very large and expensive controlled study which would probably add very little to our existing knowledge. Following a contaminated procedure, e.g. cleaning up after an incontinent patient, bacterial counts of up to $10^7$ may be isolated from washings from the hands of the attendant. The reductions obtainable even with alcohol may be inadequate and gloves should be worn for such procedures.

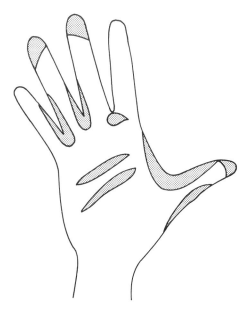

**Figure 15** Areas commonly missed with poor handwashing technique (▨). Demonstration of poor handwashing technique by use of dye

The average time of handwashing varies between 10 and 20 seconds and a thorough wash covering all surfaces is important. In a study of blindfolded nurses handwashing with a dye, certain areas were commonly missed[32] (Figure 15). A suitable technique has been described[33] to ensure adequate coverage of hands.

Nurses wash their hands much less frequently than expected and efforts are continually made to improve the frequency. However, it is not known whether this would influence the infection rate and too much washing will damage the skin.

Assessment of indications for handwashing will provide practical guidelines, although it is accepted some discrepancies will occur. Studies in our laboratory have shown that significant hand contamination with patient strains is infrequent following contact with furniture, taking pulse, temperatures, bed-making, etc., but may occur following care of incontinent patients, emptying urine bags, bedpans, etc., or after bed-bathing or handling bedding from infected or colonized patients (Table 9).

**Table 9 Pathogens on nurses' hands after ward procedures and after washing with chlorhexidine detergent**

| Procedure | Number of hands sampled | Number of hands showing | | | |
|---|---|---|---|---|---|
| | | Staph. aureus | | Gram-negative bacilli | |
| | | Before washing | After washing | Before washing | After washing |
| Dressing change | 11 | 5 | 1 | 0 | 0 |
| Bed-making | 10 | 1 | 0 | 0 | 0 |
| Bed-bathing | 15 | 6 | 1 | 1 | 1 |
| Handling bedpans | 29 | 12 | 1 | 4 | 1 |

Washing with soap and water should be sufficient for most procedures, but an antiseptic detergent may be preferred in special units or during outbreaks. Alcohol disinfection provides additional protection and can be introduced during outbreaks or where rapid disinfection is required, e.g. during rounds of patients, particularly when handwashing facilities are inadequate. The thoroughness of application is more important than the time spent on washing or the agent used.

## Aseptic techniques

Many procedures are defined as aseptic techniques, e.g. catheterization, tracheal suction, wound dressings, etc. Usually this implies the use of sterile equipment, avoidance of direct contact with the susceptible site and other measures to reduce the probability of introducing potential pathogens into a susceptible site. Procedures may vary widely from one hospital to another though attempts to standardize them have been made. Remaining differences may be due to financial restraint or personal preference but procedures should be rational, each step should be justifiable and techniques should be kept up to date taking full account of any relevant research.

*Wound dressings*

The most commonly used aseptic technique is a wound dressing. Wounds can be divided into two main categories, surgical and traumatic. The main difference between these is that surgical wounds are usually produced under carefully controlled conditions intended to prevent the access of microbes and are then carefully closed under the same conditions. The traumatic wound may be heavily contaminated with organisms at the time of injury and may contain extraneous foreign matter and dead tissue likely to encourage subsequent infection. Burns are perhaps an exception for, though clearly traumatic, they are likely to be initially sterile but because of a large area of damaged skin readily become colonized.

Surgical sepsis is more likely to be acquired at the time of operation rather than in the ward, since it is more difficult for organisms to gain access to a closed wound. The organisms causing postoperative wound infection are more likely to be derived from the patient (autogenous) than from the operating team or the theatre environment. Drained wounds are more likely to become infected especially if an open drain is used, but there would appear to be little increase in infection risk if a 'Redivac' drain or a closed drainage system is used. It is now rare for large open or corrugated drains to be used. Infection rates are also likely to be high where there is leakage from the gut or other organs containing bacteria or where there is contact with another colonized or already infected site during the operation.

Open drains and heavily discharging wounds cause additional nursing problems. Prolonged wetting of the skin by exudate and frequent removal of dressings can damage the skin, reducing the rate of healing and increasing the likelihood of infection. As soon as exudate appears on the outer surface of the dressing it should be changed, as it will no longer prevent bacteria on the outer surface from reaching the wound, and if the wound is already infected, the moist exudate on the dressing surface will contaminate hands or other surfaces coming into contact with it. Many measures may be taken to prevent damage to the surrounding skin but traditional remedies such as oatmeal paste, etc., may merely provide additional nutrition for bacterial growth. The damage caused by constantly removing and attaching sticky tape can be reduced by taping cotton tape to the skin and tying the new dressing in place. Many specialized commercial dressings are available but it would be expensive and impractical to carry stocks of each. A representative of each type should be chosen. These dressings should, however, only be used when there is a relevant specific advantage in using that particular type of dressing for an individual patient. Colostomy bags are sometimes used as wound dressings to contain copious exudate and do have some advantages but they do not entirely overcome the problem. They require frequent emptying and this may still lead to skin damage.

Procedures may become out of date and require re-evaluation. It has long been recommended that all cleaning and bed-making should cease before wound dressings are carried out or intravenous catheters are inserted. This was intended to prevent airborne contamination of the exposed site. Although this is the preferred practice, these measures have become impractical. Changes in nursing practice mean that wound dressings are likely to be carried out at irregular intervals throughout the day and changes in domestic practice mean it is often not possible to delay cleaning procedures. Table 10 shows that even when substantial disturbance of bed linen occurs, the increase in airborne counts would be unlikely to greatly increase infection risk. In the same series of experiments, liquid culture medium was left exposed for short periods in a skin ward where large numbers of heavily contaminated skin scales are dispersed. The number of organisms recovered

**Table 10 Contamination from airborne organisms**

| Site sampled | Numbers of micro-organisms settling in 5 minutes, during | | | |
| --- | --- | --- | --- | --- |
| | Bed-making | Shaking curtains | High activity | Wet cleaning |
| Cotton gauze (60 cm²) | 19.8 | 8.4 | 27.0 | 2.4 |
| Forceps (approx. 10 cm²) | 3.3 | 1.4 | 4.5 | 0.4 |

suggested that indirect transfer on to dressing trolley surfaces or instruments by the airborne route is unlikely to be a problem. Transfer on the hands of staff is likely to be much greater.

In non-touch techniques where forceps are used to avoid skin contact with the patient or the sterile dressings, the same effect can be obtained by using a gloved hand or by inverting a plastic bag over the dressing so that it is enclosed without direct contact with the hand. These methods are easier than manipulating forceps. There are perhaps many other techniques that could be re-evaluated. It is usually taught that dressing techniques are carried out by two nurses but experience suggests the second nurse is rarely available. This may leave the nurse to adapt the technique to a one nurse dressing technique without proper knowledge of the most important infection control aspects. It would be preferable if nurses were taught a deeper understanding of the principles behind the techniques so that they could adapt them for a one nurse technique safely when required. Nurses will often leave the bedside in the middle of a dressing to wash the hands, and the wound will be exposed for a longer period than is necessary. Handwashing may not be required at that time or alcohol could be applied at the bedside.

The necessity of routine cleaning of wounds is doubtful. The exudate may have a useful antimicrobial effect and the cleaning procedure may only redistribute the organisms rather than removing them, irrespective of the method used. If cleaning is considered necessary, sterile saline is usually preferable to antiseptics as these, especially hypochlorites, may delay healing. The exposure time is also likely to be inadequate to obtain effective antibacterial action. Gloved or disinfected hands tend to be more effective than forceps for cleaning the wounds and it has been shown that little contamination of fingers occurs when using disinfected hands. Studies have previously demonstrated a significant reduction in infection when using a non-touch technique, but recent evidence shows that it can at least be modified[34].

As long as the package remains dry and intact the contents of dressing packs should remain sterile, but should be examined for evidence of damage or moisture penetration, and if these are found, the pack should be returned to the Sterile Services Department. Other items on the dressing trolley are usually single use, but the inner surface of a roll of adhesive tape is unlikely to present a major infection problem and it would usually be acceptable to use non-sterile adhesive tape on intact skin. Lack of knowledge can easily lead to priorities being misjudged so that a great deal of time and effort is spent on the unnecessary steps at the expense of the more necessary.

There are many functions of a dressing and it is necessary to understand why the dressing is being applied in a particular instance; if it is to protect while healing takes place, the amount of padding may be important; if it is to promote healing, then a gauze dressing that will remove the growing epithelium along with the gauze is unsuitable. If the dressing is to protect against infection and prevent the organisms getting in or out, is it then sufficiently impermeable, or if the wound is discharging is it sufficiently absorbent to prevent strike through before the next dressing change? Where a patient requires surgery but has another infected site, occluding that site with an impervious dressing such as Opsite may prevent spread of the organism to the clean operation site and allow surgery to be carried out earlier than would otherwise be possible.

Not all wounds require aseptic techniques. There would seem little point in carrying out a rigorous aseptic technique on a colonized pressure sore which up to that point had been exposed, or even when dressing a surgical wound if the patient has just had a bath with the wound uncovered. The presence of dead tissue can prevent antibiotics or antiseptics reaching infecting organisms and can allow reduced oxygen tension which may allow anaerobes such as *Clostridium tetanii* to multiply. The presence of slough will also delay healing, but care is necessary in the use of desloughing agents that delay healing, e.g. Eusol. The greater the understanding of the interaction between the wound surface, the microbe and the individual patient, the more likely it becomes that the right treatment will be selected.

*Intravenous catheterization*

The intravenous insertion site is a break in the natural defences through which fluids are introduced into the circulation via a needle or cannula. Organisms can enter the circulation from a contaminated fluid or giving set, or can grow along the outer surface of the cannula.

Intravenous fluids are initially sterile but may be contaminated by the addition of medicaments. Total parenteral nutrition now plays a major role in therapy and the fluids can be an excellent culture medium. Some are relatively inhibitory, e.g. lipid solutions to microbial growth, but others allow the growth of certain Gram-negative bacilli, e.g. *Enterobacter* spp. and particularly of yeasts. Avoiding initial contamination of the fluid is of particular importance, and if additives are required they should be introduced aseptically, preferably in a laminar flow cabinet in the pharmacy. The role of in-line filters in prevention of infection remains uncertain. There is some evidence of a reduction in non-infectious phlebothrombosis, but there is little evidence that they reduce infection.

Contamination may also be introduced via injection ports. This potential hazard for introducing organisms remains controversial, but care is necessary to avoid the entry of organisms by this route. Containers of intravenous fluids are usually changed before significant growth occurs, but the giving set should be changed every 48–72 hours.

Catheter infections are usually due to skin organisms, mainly coagulase-negative staphylococci. These adhere to and colonize the inner and outer surfaces of the catheter. Many of the coagulase-negative staphylococci produce slime which protects them from antibiotics and the patients' defence mechanisms. The colonizing organisms can cause bacteraemia or local infections usually associated with thrombosis.

The introduction of a cannula requires the same precautions as a surgical operation, e.g. thorough disinfection of the site and non-touch technique. This is particularly important for long-term catheterization. The hands should be disinfected with alcohol and preferably sterile gloves should be worn. The skin of the insertion site should be disinfected with alcoholic chlorhexidine. Bandages and dressings may create moist conditions suitable for bacterial growth and a clear adhesive bacterial-impermeable, water vapour-permeable dressing may be preferred[35]. This also allows observation of the site without removing the dressing. However, some studies have shown an increase in bacterial growth under these dressings, but this may be reduced by reducing the skin flora to a low level before applying the dressing. The daily application of antiseptics or antibiotics to the insertion site has given variable results and the value remains doubtful.

Prevention of infection remains a problem and new approaches are required. A catheter surface to which organisms do not adhere, or the introduction of antimicrobial agents into the catheter material, are possibilities. However, avoiding catheterization or removal as soon as possible (or at least at 48 hours) are the best methods of preventing infection. Indications for catheterization need to be re-evaluated. Long-term control of catheterization will continue to be required and the possibility of enhancing host defence mechanisms is an alternative approach.

*Urinary catheterization* (see also p. 46)
The insertion of a urinary catheter is usually done with care, since the infection risks are well understood. However, the benefits can be lost by poor management of the catheter end drainage bag. The flutter valve prevents urine flowing from the bag to the tubing, but does not prevent urine in the tubing running back into the bladder. Generally, urimeters do not have flutter valves. The drainage bag should not be raised above bladder height without first clamping the tubing. Again, there are practical difficulties: bags are not generally supplied with clamps although one manufacturer now does so; gate clips and Spencer Wells forceps disappear. Not only nurses handle drainage bags: physiotherapists often pin bags above waist height when mobilizing the patient; domestic staff may rest the bag on the bed while cleaning the floor.

The collection of a catheter specimen of urine is simplified by incorporating a sample point in the tubing. This is not available on most urimeters. Provided a small bore needle is used, samples can be taken direct from the catheter, since the material of the catheter and sample point are similar.

A technique which is on the borderline between hygienic and aseptic is emptying of urine drainage bags. This is a task commonly allocated to junior members of staff who may not be aware of the risk to the patient. Use of drainage bags with taps has helped to reduce the incidence of urinary tract infection associated with indwelling catheters. Frequent disconnection at the catheter–bag junction was thought to be a major source of contamination. However, the taps themselves present a hazard and illustrate the point that every action has an influence on the system as a whole. If the tap is allowed to drag on the floor or is contaminated by handling, micro-organisms can track back into the urine in the bag. This acts as a culture medium. The flutter valve does not necessarily prevent urine in the tubing becoming contaminated. If the bag is raised above bladder height, contaminated urine will run back into the bladder. The use of disinfectant (chlorhexidine or hydrogen peroxide) in the drainage bag should prevent the growth of organisms, but its use remains controversial[36].

It is usual to recommend regular meatal toilet at 4–8-hourly intervals for those with indwelling catheters. It is a time-consuming, though a simple procedure and often seen as one that can be neglected if the ward is busy. Is frequent cleaning necessary? There is evidence to suggest that daily meatal toilet is adequate. Similar to emptying the bag, it is a procedure on the borderline between aseptic and hygienic. The catheter drains a 'sterile' body cavity and the equipment used is sterile, but the technique is hygienic. It is probably most conveniently done at the time of the daily bath, using pre-packed sterile equipment and freshly drawn tap water. This would not be necessary if the patient can use the ward bath, and is an example of balancing the effort involved against the size of the risk. While there may be some risk in using the bath, it is probably less than the risk of not having a bath. Whether the risk can be reduced by adding an antiseptic solution to the water is uncertain.

It is surprising so many uncertainties remain in the prevention of infection in catheterized patients. Avoiding the use of a catheter and removal as rapidly as possible from catheterized patients, remain the most certain methods of preventing or reducing infection. The use of incontinence pads rather than a catheter has been shown to reduce infection as has suprapubic drainage.

## Bathing the patient

Bathing is an important routine procedure for patient comfort and to reduce infection risk. It should, however, be carried out with care. It is better to clean towards the naturally heavily contaminated areas such as the rectum so that Gram-negative bacteria are not distributed over the rest of the body surface, though they will not survive long on an intact skin in good condition. It is always preferable to use a fresh disposable wipe and the same cloth should never be used on more than one patient without being properly washed and dried. Unless a fresh, disposable wash cloth is used each time, the patient may be microbiologically dirtier at the end of the bath than at the beginning. Gram-negative organisms die on drying. A dry skin is unlikely to be colonized by Gram-negative bacilli, but patients confined to bed tend to have moist, sweaty skin in the area under the bedclothes. If wash bowls are left wet and stacked, they act as incubators and bacteria multiply in the moisture trapped between the layers of bowls (Table 11). Therefore, bowls are contaminated even before use. Contaminated wash bowls have been implicated in an outbreak of infection.

When wards are under pressure, it is common practice not to change the water during a bed-bath, and to use the same wash cloth for all areas of the body. By the

**Table 11 Viable Gram-negative bacteria isolated from wet and dry wash bowls filled for patient bed-baths**

| No. of organisms per ml | Number of bowls sampled | |
|---|---|---|
|  | Wet | Dry |
| $10^3$ | 11(22%) | 47(94%) |
| $10^3$–$10^7$ | 39(78%) | 3  (6%) |
| Total | 50 | 50 |

end of the bath, the water is a soup of soap and bacteria. This presents a potential hazard if the patient has a break in the skin, e.g. surgical wound, wound drain, intravenous cannula.

### Oral toilet

This is a frequent and necessary procedure, but not an aseptic one. It serves as an example of a hygienic measure, and is particularly important for patients with nasogastric tubes, the unconscious, the immunosuppressed and those on broad-spectrum antibiotics. It is a hygienic rather than an aseptic technique, since it does not significantly breach the body's defences, rather it enhances them. Oral *Candida* infections are a common complication of debilitated patients. Chest infections are sometimes associated with nasogastric tubes since they breach the barrier between the oesophagus and trachea. Patients regurgitate and aspirate small quantities of stomach contents. It is important to ensure the actual feeds are not contaminated. Cleaning the mouth also stimulates production of saliva, a mild antiseptic, and removes crust and debris in which organisms can multiply. Since the mouth is not a sterile area, equipment used can be clean rather than sterile. A small risk exists for nurses carrying out oral toilet in that they may acquire a herpetic whitlow from the patient. This can be avoided by wearing gloves.

## Conclusions

Though Florence Nightingale did not subscribe to the germ theory of infection, she did recognize the importance of sound hygiene. It is, however, difficult to adopt the most sensible measures if the knowledge of hygiene is based on folklore and ritual. Nurses who choose infection control as their speciality, soon learn to recognize that learning the scientific theory behind good practice can be easier than unlearning the ritual and abandoning the prejudices. The amount of practice that is based on sound theory and has been scientifically evaluated is increasing but much ritual and prejudice remains. Some unnecessary practices have been abandoned because of financial pressures and others are being re-evaluated. The wearing of caps, masks and gowns for routine dressings has been abandoned by many hospitals as has the use of masks for deliveries and for use when handling premature babies; this has been done without increasing infection rates. We must not, however, be forced into abandoning procedures under financial pressure without first evaluating the effect. It is important to keep up to date with what has been evaluated as good practice and what has been abandoned as ritual.

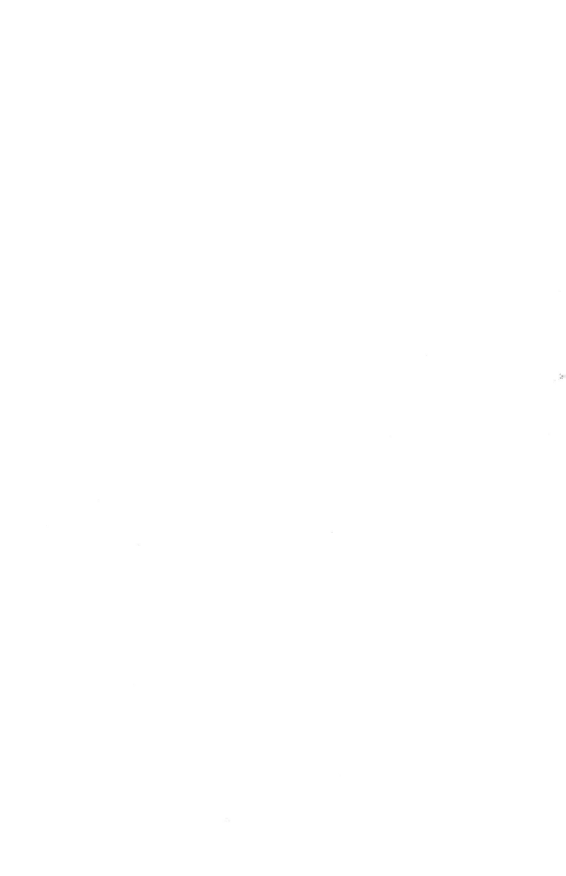

Chapter 7

# Nursing aspects of prevention of infection: isolation[37,38]

Isolation is one means by which society protects itself from those who would do it harm. Antisocial people are isolated in prison; infected people are isolated in hospital. The degree of isolation may vary between close confinement and an open prison, but whatever the degree of isolation, it is at best an unsettling experience for the person concerned.

The protection that society gains by isolating the infected has been understood since at least biblical times. Lepers were dealt with summarily. Jews in the ghettoes of Europe were protected to some degree from the plagues that ravaged the Continent by lack of contact with their Gentile neighbours.

Mechanisms for the spread of infection are now more thoroughly understood. Nevertheless, there seems to be a certain dichotomy in attitudes to those with infection. At one extreme an often irrational fear demands total isolation of the infected person, using methods which are at best of uncertain value, e.g. a suspected case of pulmonary tuberculosis screened from the ward and surrounded by a clutter of gowns hung on drip stands, laundry skip, rubbish bin, bedpan, wash bowls, crockery and cutlery soaking in hypochlorite, and a definite worry about the infection risk attached to the charts hung on the bed. At the other extreme, there is almost sublime indifference to the germ theory of disease, e.g. 'the infected wound following colonic surgery is not really an infection because it is autogeneous', therefore any wound isolation precautions are superfluous, irrespective of organisms isolated. Between these extremes lies a wealth of conjecture, guesswork, misinformation and fear of feeling foolish, most often allied to a caring, concerned attitude.

Enough information is available to develop safe isolation precautions, most of them simple enough to be practical in most wards or even in private homes, so long as there is somewhere for handwashing, a laundry and waste disposal facilities.

## When do people need isolating?

Isolation becomes necessary when a person presents an infection risk to society, when the requirement is for source isolation, i.e. containment of the source of the infection. Conversely, society itself can threaten the safety of an individual. Here the need is for protective isolation. This still means containment, but it is the community at large which presents the risk to the patient.

In either case the method for containment is the application of isolation precautions or barrier nursing. The aim is to confine the organism and block its routes of spread. This does not necessarily mean isolating the whole person, e.g. a bacteria-impermeable dressing may isolate a wound. Quite often the need for isolation can conflict with other medical or staffing problems. Nurses are reluctant to put relatively ill patients in a single room, particularly on Nightingale wards, where they feel the patient will get less than the necessary amount of attention.

Infectious diseases are relatively uncommon on general wards, more so on paediatric wards. Nevertheless, 1 in 5 patients is likely to have an infection; half of those patients will have acquired the infection in hospital. It is likely that a proportion will present a risk to the 4 out of 5 patients not infected.

The need for, and type of, isolation is related to the nature and severity of the infection, how readily it is transferred, the susceptibility of those in contact with it, the underlying reason for admission and the mobility of the patient. It also depends on having or suspecting a diagnosis of infection.

The need for isolating infectious diseases is well understood, often from an early age. Who did not appreciate the days off school because of contact with a case of measles or some other childhood disease? But the prescribed days off could be worrying if they coincided with examinations. Remembering this, it becomes easier to understand the need for a rational approach to isolation.

**Table 12 Routes of transmission and isolation precautions**

| Route | Precaution | Example |
| --- | --- | --- |
| Airborne | Respiratory | Chicken-pox, measles, whooping cough, streptococcal sore throat, tuberculosis, staphylococcal pneumonia, scarlet fever |
| | Skin | Skin disease colonized or infected by *Staph. aureus* |
| Contact | Wound | Infected discharging wounds, varicose ulcers, pressure sores |
| | Secretion/excretion | Conjunctivitis, herpes simplex and herpes zoster, urinary tract infection |
| Faecal-oral | Enteric | *Shigella, Salmonella typhi, Salmonella typhimurium*, food poisoning, enteropathogenic *E. coli*, rotavirus, hepatitis A |
| Blood | Blood | HBV (non-A, non-B), HIV infection |

Infectious diseases can be grouped according to the source and route of spread. Some of the more common reasons for isolation are summarized in Table 12 together with the appropriate isolation precautions. It can be seen that isolation precautions are based on a knowledge and understanding of the causal organism, its source and route of spread (see Chapters 2 and 3).

The first stage is to diagnose an infection, recognize the causal organism and work out its route of spread. With this information, it is possible to decide on the most appropriate form of isolation.

Isolation involves the application of a number of precautions to a specific category or disease. These precautions are grouped together in column 2 of Table 12. Brief details are summarized in Table 13. This shows the basic components of

**Table 13 Type of isolation or precautions**

| Precaution | Wound | Skin | Secretion | Blood | Enteric | Respiratory | Protective |
|---|---|---|---|---|---|---|---|
| Single room | Not usually necessary | Necessary Door shut | Not necessary | Not necessary | Desirable | Necessary Door shut | Necessary Door shut |
| Apron to be worn | Handling wound or dressings | Patient contact | Handling secretions or patient contact | Handling blood | Handling exreta | Handling secretions | Patient contact |
| Mask to be worn | No | No | No | No | No | No (or rarely) | No |
| Hands to be washed routinely | Before and after contact with infected site After contact with immediate environment | | | After contact with blood | After contact with faeces | After contact with sputum | Before and after patient contact |
| Gloves to be worn | Contact with infected site or dressing | | | Handling blood | Handling contaminated articles | | Not necessary |
| Equipment | Disposable Disinfect or sterilize | | | Disposable Disinfect or sterilize linen – water soluble or alginate stitched bags | | | Disinfect or sterilize before use |
| Comments | Isolate wound with occlusive dressing | | | Transport specimen containers in plastic bag – label 'Biohazard' | | | Exclude infected staff and visitors |

isolation and which ones are used for each isolation precaution. They are discussed in greater detail below.

Instead of categories of isolation as shown in Table 13, a system of disease-specific isolation has been proposed in the USA[39]. This is claimed to avoid over-isolation and reduce the use of unnecessary precautions in certain infections included in a broad category. Minimizing unnecessary precautions reduces costs and allows staff greater freedom in making decisions, or requirements for individual infections. A new category, contact isolation, was also introduced for most common nosocomial infections, e.g. antibiotic-resistant organisms in urinary tract infections. Our own system in which basic procedures, handwashing and wearing of plastic aprons for all patients (source and protective) requiring isolation, has the advantage of simplicity[38, 73]. Masks and gloves are rarely worn. Modifications can be made if necessary, e.g. gloves when handling bedpans of patients with *Salmonella* infection.

## Single room

A single room with the door shut is intended to prevent the transmission of organisms spread by the airborne route, and to prevent gross contamination of the environment outside of the room with certain organisms spread by contact. For this latter group of patients the door may be left open, since airborne spread is not a problem. Nevertheless, it is often difficult to define the relative importance of airborne and contact spread in many infections. Confinement to a single room can be an unpleasant experience. Whilst it is necessary to restrict the patient, it can also discourage staff from entering the room. The patient can feel deprived of human contact, therefore a single room should not be used if airborne transmission is unlikely, or if there is little risk of heavy environmental contamination. Glass partitions, speak-through panels and television sets help to reduce the feeling of isolation.

## Aprons

Transmission of organisms from clothing of staff is possible, but not a major problem (Table 14). Heavy contamination of protective clothing was uncommon in our society and Gram-negative bacilli were infrequently isolated. However, it is rational to protect uniforms when infected material is being handled. The area at waist height is most often contaminated but may extend to lower or higher levels depending on the procedure. An impermeable plastic apron offers better protection than a cotton gown, although the latter are often preferred by medical staff. It is uncommon for the shoulder area of the uniform to become contaminated, even when lifting a patient, but long sleeves should be rolled up. Plastic aprons can be used more than once for the same patient, provided the outer surface is marked, and it is kept within the room or hanging by the bed. An apron with a different colour on each side is particularly useful.

It is difficult to understand the rationale for keeping gowns hanging outside the room since this will neither contain contamination inside the room nor prevent transfer outside. If the gown is intended to prevent uniforms becoming contaminated, it does so by itself becoming contaminated. Hung outside the room,

**Table 14 Recovery of *Staph. aureus* and Gram-negative bacilli from nurses' uniforms after wearing cotton gowns or plastic aprons on an isolation ward\***

| No. of colony forming units/ contact plate 25 cm² | Cotton gowns | | Plastic aprons | |
|---|---|---|---|---|
| | Front (n=133) | Shoulder (n=118) | Front (n=166) | Shoulder (n=166) |
| *Staph. aureus* | | | | |
| 0 | 89 (66.9%) | 89 (75.4%) | 118 (71.1%) | 134 (80.7%) |
| 1–10 | 43 (32.3%) | 29 (24.6%) | 46 (23.7%) | 30 (18.1%) |
| 11–50 | 1  (0.7%) | 0 | 2  (1.2%) | 1  (0.6%) |
| 51+ | 0 | 0 | 0 | 1  (0.6%) |
| Gram-negative bacilli | | | | |
| 0 | 126 (94.7%) | 112 (94.9%) | 162 (97.6%) | 163 (98.2%) |
| 1–10 | 7  (5.3%) | 6  (5.1%) | 3  (1.8%) | 3  (1.8%) |
| 11–50 | 0 | 0 | 1  (0.6%) | 0 |
| 51+ | 0 | 0 | 0 | 0 |

\* from Babb, J. R. *et al.* (1983) *J. Hosp. Infect.* **4**, 149

it must surely present a hazard to other staff. It presents no risk to the infected patient because he already has the disease. The relative lack of evidence for the spread of infection by this route indicates the low risk of infection attached to protective clothing. However, clothing may transfer staphylococci from the rooms of heavy dispersers.

# Masks

At one time it was common practice to wear masks for many ward procedures. It is now recognized that this practice contributes little to patient or staff safety on the wards. The results from a prevalence survey in the West Midlands are shown in Table 15[22]. The wound infection rate was not obviously influenced by the wearing of masks and protective clothing for carrying out wound dressings. The rationale

**Table 15 Protective clothing and wound sepsis (cross-sectional surveys of infection in hospitals in West Midlands)[22]**

| | Number wearing no additional protective clothing | Type of protective clothing worn in wards | | | | |
|---|---|---|---|---|---|---|
| | | Mask | Gown | Mask and gown | Gown, mask and cap | Total |
| Total patients in group | 675 | 1196 | 84 | 656 | 236 | 2847 |
| No. of infected wounds | 77 (11.41%) | 192 (16.05%) | 12 (14.29%) | 121 (18.45%) | 34 (14.41%) | 436 (15.31%) |

for wearing a mask is either to protect the patient from the staff or the staff from the patient. If the nurse has a cold, a sore throat or influenza, she should be off duty, not wearing a mask. *Staph. aureus* is unlikely to be dispersed in the air in large numbers directly from the nose of a carrier. It is more likely to be spread by improper use of a mask, i.e. handling the mask, followed by handling the patient without washing the hands first. Masks are no substitute for good technique and careful handwashing, There is an area of uncertainty as regards the use of masks by staff dressing burns or large open wounds, and for certain procedures, e.g. lumbar puncture, bone marrow biopsy. Whilst there is no great evidence that use of a mask contributes to preventing infection in these circumstances, some authorities may still recommend their use. Every nurse should be immune to tuberculosis and diphtheria. A mask is therefore superfluous, although some may prefer to wear one in close contact with open, untreated pulmonary tuberculosis. However, there may be some logic in requesting that the patient wears a mask. As regards the common childhood fevers, non-immune nurses should not be allowed to care for such patients. There may be some reason for wearing a mask during the first 48 hours of specific treatment for meningococcal meningitis, although by the time a bacteriological diagnosis is made it may be rather late to do so and there is little evidence of spread to hospital staff. Specific antibiotic prophylaxis is more appropriate. Masks are therefore rarely required for nursing patients in source or protective isolation. However, if a mask is thought to be necessary, it should be an efficient filter type.

## Handwashing

As already stated in Chapter 6, handwashing is the most important method of preventing the spread of infection by contact.

In our study on an isolation ward, there was no cross-infection when non-medicated bar soap, chlorhexidine-detergent or 70% alcohol was used. Bacterial counts showed little difference (Table 16) between the three regimes although Gram-negative bacilli were less after the use of 70% alcohol. It is more important to ensure hands are actually washed or disinfected than to worry about the choice of agents.

**Table 16 Influence of soap and antiseptics on the transient hand carriage of nurses in an isolation ward**

| | Percentage of samples | | | | | |
| --- | --- | --- | --- | --- | --- | --- |
| | Chlorhexidine-detergent | | Bar soap | | 70% alcohol | |
| Range of cfu* per sample | Staph. aureus | GNB** | Staph. aureus | GNB | Staph. aureus | GNB |
| 1 000 000 | 0 | 0 | 0 | 2 | 0 | 0 |
| 10 000–1 000 000 | 5 | 10 | 4 | 12 | 8 | 1 |
| 200–10 000 | 12 | 11 | 8 | 9 | 13 | 2 |
| < 200 | 83 | 79 | 88 | 77 | 79 | 97 |

* cfu = colony forming units
** GNB = Gram-negative bacilli

# Gloves

Gloves may be used for several reasons: to prolong the effect of hand disinfection; to reduce gross contamination of the hands from infected sites or equipment, thus reducing the number of organisms to be removed by handwashing; to protect the patient from the nurse's normal flora or transient flora; to facilitate manipulation of sterile equipment. In any event, the use of a glove does not remove the need for handwashing. It is important to wear gloves when handling material contaminated with large numbers of organisms. Handwashing alone may not be sufficient.

Gloves are increasingly worn for handling materials due to the potential but unknown hazard of HIV infections. The Centres for Disease Control recommend 'universal' precautions for contact with blood or blood-stained fluids from any patient. This has considerably increased the cost of patient management.

If the incidence of HIV is low it may not be considered necessary to wear gloves for taking blood other than from high risk patients. This will depend on the skill of the operator. It is still advisable to wear gloves when cleaning up blood-stained spillage. Consideration should also be given to the type of glove and whether it is intact prior to use.

# Overshoes

Contamination of floors is discussed in Chapter 8. In operating theatres where patients are particularly vulnerable and contamination needs to be kept to a minimum, it is rational to wear different shoes within the theatre suite. However there is no such requirement in isolation nursing. The floor is not a source of infection so long as the patients are nursed in bed and equipment that falls to the floor is decontaminated before re-use. In one reported incident the probable cause of an outbreak of *Pseudomonas* infection in a renal unit was the use of overshoes. Persons entering the unit were required to wear overshoes. In putting them on, the hands were contaminated with *Pseudomonas* from the floor. Patients and equipment were then handled without adequate handwashing. The method of spread was clearly by contact associated with poor handwashing, but this was secondary to the unnecessary use of overshoes. Any *Pseudomonas* would otherwise have stayed harmlessly on the floor. This outbreak illustrates two points:

1. If an organism is doing no harm, leave it alone; and
2. Protective clothing does not prevent contact spread nor does it compensate for a lack of professional self-discipline.

# Equipment

Equipment as a source and route of spread of infection is discussed in Chapter 8. Whether a patient is being isolated or not, equipment must always be sterilized or properly decontaminated before use. When infection occurs, certain pieces of equipment may present a somewhat greater risk depending on the site of infection and the route of spread. For example, respiratory equipment, oral thermometers, crockery and cutlery during a respiratory tract infection; bedpans or urinals are no more of a problem than for any other patient, apart from some virus infections affecting both the respiratory and gastrointestinal tracts.

## Crockery and cutlery

These may present some risk after use by patients on blood, enteric, respiratory or secretion precautions, if the infection is in the mouth. Decontamination in a dishwasher with a final rinse temperature of 80°C is the method of choice (Chapter 12). Washing by hand may be inadequate. An acceptable alternative to a dishwasher is disposable crockery and cutlery, although patients may find this unacceptable. Anyone who has eaten food in an aircraft can readily appreciate their feelings.

Quite often the diagnosis is made after the patient has been in hospital for some days. Lack of evidence for spread by this route may indicate that it is relatively unimportant. Nevertheless, a severe infection, such as typhoid, may still cause anxiety.

## Bathing

The bath is unlikely to be a route of spread of respiratory infection, but may be so with enteric, wound or skin infection. Patients with infected lesions on wound precautions or with a urinary tract infection on secretion/excretion precautions may benefit from the addition of a disinfectant to the bath water, e.g. povidone-iodine. Patients on skin precautions, where *Staph. aureus* rather than Gram-negative bacteria are the main problem, may benefit more from the use of chlorhexidine detergent applied directly to the skin, then washed off. Salt is often added to bath water. Whatever else salt does, it does not disinfect bath water. The bath should be cleaned with a non-abrasive hypochlorite powder before use (to remove contamination from the previous occupant), and after bathing (to remove contamination from the infected patient). Bath water contains large numbers of micro-organisms which are redistributed over the skin and contaminate the towel and environment. Showers are preferable.

Patient wash bowls have been implicated in at least one ward outbreak of infection. A bowl that is inadequately decontaminated before use will still be contaminated by organisms from the previous patient. The organisms most likely to be found are Gram-negative bacteria. Cleaning and thorough drying will reduce their numbers to below the level of an infecting dose.

## Caps

It is difficult to understand the rationale for the use of caps outside the operating theatre. There may be a slight possibility of some transient carriage of *Staph. aureus* on the hair, acquired from a patient with skin disease, possibly during bed-making when large numbers of organisms are dispersed. Provided the hair is kept clean and tidy, this would seem to be a minimal risk, not justifying the use of caps. If a member of staff has a skin lesion, including one of the scalp, this requires treatment and possibly sick leave, not the use of protective clothing.

## Needles and sharp instruments ('sharps')

'Sharps' require safe disposal at all times, but especially after use on hepatitis carriers and patients with HIV infection (see p. 117). Additional precautions are not generally required, although it is worth noting that most injuries to laundry handlers are from 'sharps'. Porters removing waste are particularly at risk from needles inadvertently discarded into plastic bags.

## Specimens

Laboratory staff are at risk of acquiring infection, since they handle material from infected patients and may well make the first diagnosis of infection. However, the incidence of laboratory-acquired infection is low. Portering staff are also at some slight risk from contamination of the outside of specimen containers, especially sputum specimens. If an infection likely to infect the staff is suspected, or already diagnosed, specimens from the infected site should be transported in plastic bags and clearly labelled 'Biohazard'.

## Charts

Charts are handled by a variety of people. It is therefore often assumed that they present a greater infection hazard than is in fact the case. Charts are usually clean and dry, and therefore unlikely to support survival of pathogens. There is some logic in keeping them outside the room, since this discourages quick visits to the room, possibly leading to a break in isolation techniques.

## Mattress covers and duvets

In general, mattress and pillow covers can be adequately decontaminated by the physical action of cleaning with detergent and water. Guidelines issued by the DHSS prevent the use of duvets which do not meet stringent fire regulations, except when there is an overriding clinical need, e.g. rheumatology units. However, a duvet designed for hospital use, and which meets the fire regulations, is now available. This has a waterproof cover. It does not require laundering, but is decontaminated by wiping with a detergent. Phenolics may damage the waterproof fabric, therefore a hypochlorite or 70% alcohol can be used as an alternative if disinfection is required. However, there can be problems of patient acceptability with impervious duvet covers. It is more usual to enclose the duvet in a fabric cover. Providing the cover does not become wet or heavily soiled, this may be acceptable as an alternative.

## Visitors

Generous visiting times often lead to claims of increased infection rates. It is difficult to understand how properly supervised visitors can be any more of a risk than properly supervised staff, although it is easy to see that some visitors can be difficult to supervise. Visitors should observe the same precautions as staff, whether on a general ward or when isolation precautions are in force. This means excluding people with an infectious disease or an infected lesion which is not properly covered. If the patient has an infectious disease, anyone not immune to that disease should not be admitted.

## Protective isolation (see also p. 125)

This is a reversal of the methods used for source isolation, hence the alternative title 'reverse barrier nursing'. It is used for patients who, because of disease or drugs, have reduced immunological competence and are therefore susceptible to infection from a lower infecting dose than in health, and possibly from organisms which are not usually pathogenic.

Potential sources are other patients and staff. Since they cannot be isolated, the patient is protected by reversing the isolation precautions. Equipment and linen leaving the room, and the room itself, do not present an infection risk any greater than if it had been used for any other patient.

## Priorities for isolation

Several factors can influence the practicality of carrying out isolation precautions. These include the availability of a single room, the mix of patients in a ward or unit, staffing levels, general facilities, such as wash hand basins and a bedpan washer or macerator, availability of staff trained in isolation techniques and the overall condition of the patient

To ensure that the salient points of isolation precautions are not missed, whatever the circumstances, a number of questions need to be asked. What is the route by which the infection spreads? Does this present a real risk to other patients, relatives and staff? Will there be any additional risk to the patient if isolation precautions are instituted? Which of these two risks is greater? Which isolation precaution is indicated? Does it need any modification due to the patient's condition or the facilities available?

In some instances (open pulmonary tuberculosis is an example) the need for isolation is self-evident. In other instances, such as an infected, profusely discharging wound, the need may be less obvious. If a single room is available, there may be other priorities for its use, e.g. a disruptive or terminally ill or private patient. Often there are no easy answers. Decisions must be made to meet the circumstances prevailing at the time, but the decisions should be based on the interest of the individual patient, the interests of the ward at large and sometimes the interests of the community. Any decision should be based on sound information.

Isolation precautions are the minimum requirements necessary to prevent the spread of infection. There is little room for the personal preferences of staff. The safety of all concerned depends on compliance with these minimal requirements. Each person has a duty to the individual patient, to other patients on the ward or unit and to professional colleagues, not to break the rules without good evidence for doing so. The essentials are good handwashing, possibly a protective apron and adequate decontamination of equipment for both source and protective isolation.

# Chapter 8

# The hospital environment

The hospital environment includes all structures, fixtures, fittings, furnishings, equipment and supplies contained within its boundaries. The microbial ecology of the environment is influenced by the persons present and their activities. Responsibility for ensuring that these activities do not put the community at risk should be extended to include materials and patients transferred from the hospital environment to the community.

Any environment can be an infection risk to specific highly susceptible individuals. The requirement to prevent environmental contamination should not be greater for hospitals than any other premises except where it is known that a specific risk exists, or where a patient is vulnerable to a level of microbial contamination that would normally be acceptable in the community.

To control infection it may be necessary to minimize, reduce or eliminate microbial contamination in any part of the environment. The need to do so should be considered at the earliest possible stage when changes in structures or procedures are planned and when the purchase of new equipment is being considered. It may be more difficult and more expensive to make major changes at a later stage.

Microbial decontamination may involve cleaning, disinfection or sterilization, and may include destructive methods such as incineration. Each of these methods is likely to be progressively more expensive and destructive and must be chosen with care, relating cost to the risk of transferring infection.

To choose the most appropriate method of decontamination some knowledge of the specific routes and sources of infection is necessary. Consultation between the user, the person responsible for the decontamination procedure and a member of the Infection Control Team is desirable.

Control measures should be based on sound principles and can be summarized as follows:

1. The environment should be hostile to the multiplication of pathogens, e.g. clean, dry, exposed to light, and well ventilated.
2. Susceptible sites on patients or susceptible patients should be protected from significant contamination, e.g. by a suitable dressing for a wound or by separating the infected from the susceptible patient in an isolation ward.
3. The resistance of the susceptible host should be increased where possible or relevant, e.g. hepatitis B vaccine to staff in a drug addiction unit.
4. 'Infectious' materials should be adequately contained and decontaminated to prevent subsequent transfer of infection.

Consideration of these principles can assist in the identification of potentially high risk situations; examples are listed below:

1. Pathogens may grow where there is spillage of blood, pus, urine, vomit or faeces, unless it is removed promptly and both the spillage and cleaning materials are disposed of safely.
2. Raw meat, waste food, used cleaning materials or wet equipment are usually heavily contaminated with Gram-negative bacilli which may consist of intestinal pathogens or opportunistic organisms, e.g. *Ps. aeruginosa.*
3. Bathrooms, toilets and sluice rooms are associated with moist conditions and are often badly ventilated. These conditions may be conducive to the survival of Gram-negative bacilli.
4. Equipment likely to come into contact with a break in the skin or mucous membranes, or to be inserted into sterile areas such as the bladder, require sterilization, e.g. dressings, surgical instruments, sutures, catheters and parenteral fluids.
5. Materials that have been in contact with specific infections may require particular care in handling, transporting and disposal, e.g. soiled dressings or linen, secretions and excretions.
6. The immediate environment of a patient suffering from an unusually virulent infection or a specified communicable disease may require additional decontamination measures to ensure it is safe for re-use by another patient.
7. Additional resources may be required to make the immediate environment safe for use by a highly susceptible patient, e.g. units for the treatment of leukaemics and other heavily immunosuppressed patients, operating theatres, intensive care units and special care baby units.

Structural surfaces, e.g. walls and floors, furniture, fixtures and fittings are unlikely to come into prolonged or intimate contact with a susceptible site and are a low infection risk. These surfaces rarely require more than periodic cleaning. Pathogens are unlikely to be present in sufficient number to cause infection or, if present, to reach a susceptible site on the patient.

In high risk situations more frequent cleaning may be required and surfaces, furnishings and fittings should be chosen which are easy to clean and will withstand frequent and thorough cleaning without excessive deterioration. The complete removal of all microbes is not practical or desirable except for 'high risk' items such as surgical instruments.

The unnecessary use of chemical disinfectants, harsh cleaning materials, or even excessive water can shorten the life of environmental surfaces. An example is the frequent cleaning of mattress covers with phenolic disinfectants which may damage the waterproofing and allow moisture to penetrate, enabling *Ps. aeruginosa* to grow in the foam under the cover. These organisms may then spread from the mattress to lesions on patients subsequently occupying the bed. Disinfectants have also been responsible for erosion of terrazzo floors and the hardening and discoloration of plastic floor finishes. Excessive use of water which penetrates floor joints and coverings may provide sufficient trapped moisture to allow bacteria to grow under the flooring material causing subsequent damage to the underlying structure. Disinfectants may also exert a selective influence on the microbial population. Outbreaks of infection caused by *Ps. aeruginosa* and *Serratia marcescens* have occurred in intensive care units possibly due to use of concentrations of disinfectants to which these organisms are resistant, allowing them to reach unusually high numbers.

Bacteria cannot grow or survive for long periods on clean dry surfaces and disinfection of structural surfaces, furniture, fixtures and fittings is rarely required except following soiling by potentially infectious material, e.g. blood, pus, faeces or urine, from patients with transmissible infections. In high risk areas the need to select material capable of withstanding frequent and thorough decontamination may conflict with appearance or patient comfort. This, however, is not a problem in all clinical areas and a balance between infection risk, appearance and practical considerations must be achieved.

## Air

The number of organisms present in air within a room will depend on the number of people occupying the room, their activity and the rate at which the air is replaced (Figure 16). Bacteria recovered from air samples consist mainly of Gram-positive cocci originating from the skin of the occupants. Pathogens represent less than 1% of the total, and of these *Staph. aureus* is the most likely. *Staph. aureus* can reach large numbers if dispersed from a patient with an infected lesion, or particularly from an infected exfoliative skin condition, but since the contaminated skin scales are relatively heavy they will not usually remain suspended in the air for long periods. Droplets projected from the infected upper respiratory tract may contain a wide variety of organisms, and some infections can be spread by this route, e.g. colds, influenza, childhood infectious diseases and tuberculosis, but an infective dose, with some exceptions, is rarely carried more than a few feet before the droplets settle or the organisms die. However, some bacteria (e.g. tubercle bacilli) or viruses may remain viable in dried droplets (droplet nuclei) and can be transported for considerable distances. Gram-negative bacteria only tend to be found in the air when associated with aerosols from contaminated fluids from humidifiers and tend to die on drying. However, spread can sometimes occur over relatively long distances e.g. *Legionella* from cooling towers.

In exceptional circumstances, other skin-associated bacteria, e.g. *Staph. epidermidis,* can cause infection, but their source especially in hospital wards is

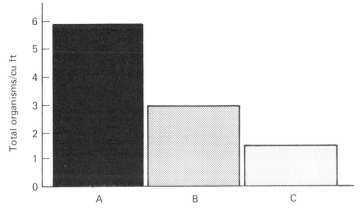

**Figure 16** Counts of airborne bacteria. A, window ventilation (5 air changes/hour); B, partial recirculation (10 air changes/hour); C, plenum ventilation (20 air changes/hour)

more likely to be autogenous transfer from the patient's own skin to an intravascular catheterization site.

Mechanical ventilation of wards or ward dressing stations may be required for comfort but is unlikely to reduce infection rates. The 20 air changes per hour normally provided in ventilated operating theatres is sufficient for most general surgery and is probably required more to improve comfort than to reduce infection risk. The provision of ultra clean air can be of value in joint replacement or other implant surgery and may be of value where large incisions remain exposed for long periods, e.g. cardiovascular surgery, but there is no evidence to justify the additional expense for routine surgery. Nevertheless, an improved method of ventilation should be possible to provide maximum protection at the wound site. The use of an isolator is a possible method, but is often cumbersome or impractical.

*Aspergillus fumigatus* and occasionally other fungal spores may cause an invasive infection in severely immunocompromised patients. It is normally present in the air and is particularly likely to be transmitted during building operations in or close to the hospital. Prevention requires high level air filtration.

## Influence of design

The microbial population of any enclosed space can be influenced by design. An adequate air flow will help to remove microbes as they are shed. If the room is inhabited, little can be achieved by temperature control since human pathogens tend to survive well at any temperature in the range acceptable to people. Moisture control is more important since most microbes multiply readily in a moist environment. The provision of surfaces which can easily be kept clean and dry and on which soil or spillage is readily seen and removed will therefore reduce infection risk. Bacteria-carrying particles tend to settle on horizontal surfaces and will not readily adhere to smooth vertical surfaces. Unnecessary horizontal surfaces, heavily textured moisture-retaining surfaces, and any inaccessible areas where moisture or soil may accumulate should therefore be avoided in patient treatment areas. However, even inappropriate surfaces are unlikely to be a major infection hazard and in most areas other factors such as cost or aesthetic appearance may be more relevant.

## Floors and other horizontal surfaces

Bacteria shed by patients and staff will usually be dispersed as droplets from the respiratory tract or as skin scales, and will tend to be carried on particles more than $10\,\mu m$ in diameter. Bacteria-carrying particles shed by infected patients and their immediate surroundings, e.g. from clothing and bedding, are the greatest risk. In reasonably still air these particles will settle fairly rapidly onto horizontal surfaces, usually the floor. After deposition they will tend to remain unless disturbed. The number of bacteria present on the floor of a busy 30-bedded ward may be quite high, e.g. between 1000 and 2000 cfu per $100\,cm^2$. The predominant organisms are likely to be *Staph. epidermidis* and *Bacillus* spp., other coagulase-negative cocci and diphtheroids present on shed skin scales. These organisms make up about 99% of the total on a dry ward floor. The only potential pathogens commonly found are *Staph. aureus* and *Clostridium welchii*. Infection risk is small. *Staph. epidermidis*

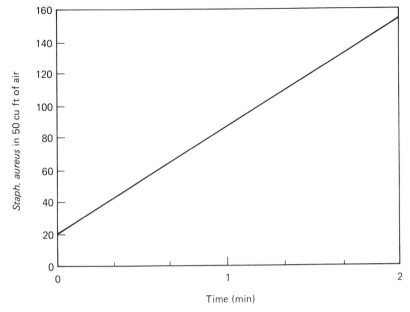

**Figure 17** Increase in airborne count of *Staphylococcus aureus* during sweeping

and diphtheroids from inanimate surfaces rarely cause infections. *Staph. aureus* and *Clostridium* spp., although capable of causing infections, are not likely to reach a susceptible site in sufficient numbers to cause infection unless vigorously redistributed into the air, e.g. by sweeping with a broom (Figure 17). Even then, the evidence of hazard is doubtful, particularly with clostridia. Normal movement and air currents have little influence on airborne counts and different types of hard flooring show only minor differences[6].

The behaviour of organisms on soft flooring such as carpets is different, but if properly managed does not increase infection risks[41]. Gram-negative bacteria are rare in a dry environment. Their presence is often associated with recent wet cleaning or fluid spillage, but they tend to disappear rapidly as the surface dries (see Chapter 2). Some organisms may survive for longer periods if protected by layers of grease or protein from blood, urine or other secretions.

In hospital wards, microbial counts from floors tend to remain remarkably static throughout the day, cleaning and disinfection having only a temporary effect on numbers. This is because bacteria tend to be shed at a fairly constant rate by the same group of individuals occupying the same ward. Factors which affect the rate of dying of bacteria are also reasonably constant, e.g. temperature, light and humidity. Cleaning will rapidly reduce numbers of bacteria on a floor. Wet cleaning with a detergent can reduce counts by about 80%. The use of a disinfectant can further increase the reduction to 95–99%[42]. However, these organisms are rapidly replaced from continuing dispersal by the occupants of the room and a plateau is reached in which an equilibrium between deposition and death or removal occurs.

The time taken to establish this equilibrium after cleaning can be as short as 2 hours in a large busy ward (Figure 18). While the use of a disinfectant instead of a

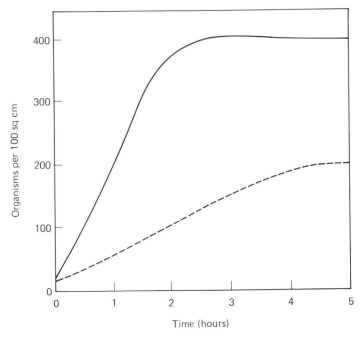

**Figure 18** Recontamination of floors after cleaning: —— surgical ward; ‑‑‑‑ operating theatre

detergent can increase the reduction in numbers of bacteria by up to 20%, the effect of the additional reduction is so transient that the disadvantages may outweigh the advantages. The disinfectant may cause injury to the operator, will add cost, possibly increase damage to the surface, may leave behind undesirable residues and can promote a false sense of security. Disinfectants are not, therefore, recommended for routine cleaning. Occasionally a patient with abnormal skin, e.g. eczema or psoriasis, which becomes colonized with *Staph. aureus*, may disperse large numbers of these organisms on skin scales. These patients, i.e. dispersers, may be a substantial risk to others with unhealed wounds and should be identified and isolated, although dispersal directly from the patient is a greater risk than redispersal from the floor. Nevertheless, it is sensible to try to eliminate the pathogens in known contaminated spillage more rapidly and completely by using a disinfectant although it is doubtful if the risk of transfer is greatly reduced. Results obtained from a large survey showed that the regular use of disinfectants for floor cleaning had no significant effect on wound infection or the nasal acquisition rate of *Staph. aureus*[22].

If it is considered necessary to reduce the height of the plateau of organisms on the floor surface it can be achieved either by reducing the number of occupants in the room or increasing the frequency of cleaning. In the example shown in Figure 18, hourly cleaning would be required to reduce the level by 50% and this is obviously not practical. Increasing the rate of air flow would remove some particles before they settled but the small particles may remain suspended longer, possibly increasing the likelihood of reaching a susceptible site.

Accumulation of soil in cracks, joints and corners is unpleasant but there is little evidence that this is a cause of infection. However, joints should be avoided if possible; if unavoidable, wall junctions and joints should be welded or sealed. This prevents an accumulation of bacteria-containing debris and fluids seeping under the surface. Plastic or carpet tiles, even when well laid, often shrink and expose open joints.

# Walls and ceilings

Bacteria-containing particles do not readily adhere to walls or attach to ceilings, but may do so if the surface becomes moist, sticky or damaged. Excessive cleaning and the use of harsh chemicals can damage surfaces to the extent that the adhesion of bacteria becomes more likely. However, there is little evidence that walls and ceilings cause infection, even if damaged or contaminated. Bacterial counts from intact wall surfaces are unlikely to exceed one or two colony forming units (cfu) per 10 sq cm and tests carried out in an operating theatre showed no evidence of a build-up over a 3-month period[6]. These findings have now been confirmed over a 6-month period.

Splashes should be cleaned immediately, particularly if they consist of excreta or material known to be contaminated with potential pathogens. Routine cleaning of ward walls at a frequency greater than once a year cannot be justified on microbiological evidence. More frequent cleaning of the walls of operating theatres (every 6 months) and pharmacy clean rooms may be considered desirable, but even in these areas there is little evidence that more frequent cleaning will reduce the numbers of bacteria on the wall or influence the airborne count. Smooth impervious finishes are preferred in patient treatment areas since they are easier to clean and bacteria will not readily adhere to them, but it is doubtful if, where textured surfaces have been installed, this will greatly increase the infection risk. The space above false ceilings may allow dust to accumulate and can provide harbourage for pests. Where provided, this space should be checked on completion of building to ensure that it has been left clean and not used for discarding unwanted materials and it should also be checked to ensure that there is no access for birds and other pests. Perforated ceilings and removable tiles may allow dust to fall on to the area below, particularly if disturbed during maintenance work. This type of ceiling is probably undesirable in operating rooms and treatment areas.

# Fixtures and fittings

Fixtures and fittings should be well designed so that they are easy to clean and do not accumulate dirt or 'soil'. Electric points and switches will probably be wet cleaned and should be of the type that will not allow moisture penetration. All fittings should be listed and included in cleaning schedules.

### Sinks, wash-basins and drains

Sinks and wash-basins should be either sealed to the wall or sufficiently far from the wall to allow cleaning of all surfaces. Where sinks are used for emptying cleaning fluids, a splash-back should be fitted to allow cleaning and prevent wall damage.

**Table 17 Isolation of *Ps. aeruginosa* from 116 wash-basins in a general hospital**

| Site | Positive (no.) | Isolates (%) |
|---|---|---|
| Outlet and grill | 6 | 5.2 |
| Fluid from trap | 27 | 23.2 |

Taps that cause splashing from a shallow sink or discharge directly into the drain hole may disperse contaminated aerosols. Sink outlets and U-bends are commonly colonized with Gram-negative bacteria (Table 17). Overflows are difficult to clean and rapidly become contaminated and should be avoided in high risk areas as they may become reservoirs of epidemic strains of Gram-negative bacilli. Where they already exist, there is little justification in taking expensive measures unless there is definite evidence of transfer of infection from the sink to the patient. Disinfection of sink traps is rarely necessary as a routine and is difficult to achieve. Although heated sink traps are effective these should not be necessary[43]. Parts that may become colonized with epidemic strains should be easy to remove, clean and replace.

## Water supply

Mains water is usually of a good bacteriological quality and contains very few bacteria. Hypochlorites are usually added by the water authority and kept at a carefully controlled level sufficient to prevent any bacterial multiplication. When this water is stored in tanks, contamination from algae, protozoa, insects, dead birds or droppings may neutralize the hypochlorite. If this occurs the small number of bacteria present may then multiply to reach large numbers. While many of the organisms present are not recognized pathogens and rarely cause infection they can contaminate equipment and could cause infection in very susceptible patients. Bulk water storage tanks should be examined at intervals and if necessary cleaned and/or chlorinated. Checking, and replacement of lids if necessary, is also important. Heating water and allowing it to cool may also dechlorinate it, and water standing unused in lengths of pipe or trapped in tap washers may produce an increase in bacterial counts. Despite these problems, tap water is very rarely an infection risk to the healthy person. These problems may be particularly relevant to Legionnaires' disease (see p. 37). Since the organism is often associated with growth of algae and protozoa, thorough cleaning of static tanks once or twice a year is advisable. Cooling towers should be cleaned at the beginning and end of the summer season, but continuous chlorination may only be required if clinical problems exist. An improved design for cooling towers avoiding aerosol production is advised on new buildings.

Showers are obviously only a small risk considering the number of people showering every day. Care should be taken if showers are used at infrequent intervals, and especially if used by compromised patients. A shower head designed to eliminate static water may be advisable in units for immunosuppressed patients. Where possible and when replacements are required appropriate fittings, e.g. plastic washers, etc., should be used which do not support the growth of *Legionella*.

# Furniture

Furniture is a minor infection risk but should have, as far as possible, a readily cleanable surface, an impervious finish, be free from ledges which may accumulate dust or retain moisture which may become contaminated from spilled urine, etc. (Figure 19). It should be positioned and designed to prevent dust and dirt accumulating in inaccessible areas below or behind it and it should be possible to clean it with available equipment. Upholstered chairs with foam filling and permeable covers may be unsuitable for incontinent patients. The foam may become contaminated with urine, allowing Gram-negative bacteria to grow and act as a reservoir for infection, and unpleasant smells.

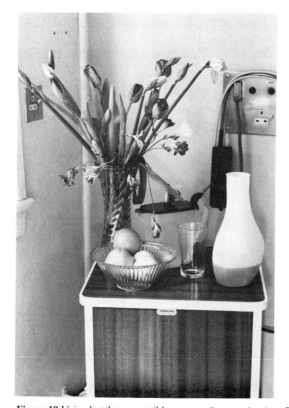

**Figure 19** Urine bottles as possible source of contamination. Flowers are an unlikely source

Mattress and pillow covers described as waterproof rapidly become pervious when subjected to regular cleaning. The manufacturers should be consulted on suitable methods of decontamination and if covers cannot be cleaned by suitable methods they should not be purchased. They should be examined at intervals, and stained or worn areas should be checked to ensure they are not impermeable and likely to contaminate the underlying mattress.

# Medical equipment

Medical equipment is often brought into close contact with a susceptible site on the patient and infection can be transferred if the equipment has not been properly decontaminated after previous use. The required method should be determined before the equipment is purchased. A cheap item that needs regular treatment by an expensive method is not necessarily more economical if costed over its period of use. Equipment that can be decontaminated by readily available means should be given priority providing it is suitable for its purpose. Equipment should be cleaned and dried, tanks and reservoirs should be emptied before storage to prevent the growth of Gram-negative bacilli.

## Anaesthetic and respiratory equipment[44]

Many ventilators and anaesthetic machines are difficult to clean as it is usually impossible to gain access to the circuits without considerable skill, time and effort. Autoclavable circuits are available and should be used on known infectious patients, e.g those with tuberculosis. Machines can be protected from contamination in use by appropriate filters[40, 45]. Decontamination with formalin gas or nebulized hydrogen peroxide is possible but difficult, and methods should be carefully evaluated before deciding whether they are suitable for any particular model. Chemicals can damage internal finishes and may cause valves to block or stick. Disinfectants can also be neutralized or deposited on the walls of the circuit before they have penetrated its entire length. A valve or bypass which opens in use and becomes contaminated may remain closed during the decontamination process. Bacteria remaining in this site may then multiply and although all parts of the circuit tested after decontamination are apparently free from organisms, subsequent re-growth may infect the next patient[46]. Infections caused by this mechanism are difficult to detect and probably very rare but can occur. *Ps. aeruginosa* is a common contaminant of respiratory equipment. Healthy people can inhale very large numbers of these organisms without apparent harm, but when forced directly into the already damaged respiratory system of the ventilated patient, they can, and do, cause infection. The mask connectors, rebreathing bag and corrugated tubing connecting a patient to an anaesthetic machine or ventilator are subjected to a flow of moist, contaminated, expired air. The moisture accumulates and allows the bacteria to grow. Viruses may also survive in these conditions. Substantial bacterial growth may occur overnight in anaesthetic equipment. It is not always practical to provide each anaesthetized patient with a fresh set but when used for a patient with an infectious disease known to be spread by this route, e.g. tuberculosis, the set should be immediately removed and autoclaved or disposable equipment should be used.

It can be seen from Table 18 that providing a fresh set for each operating session will substantially reduce the risk[47]. The small numbers of organisms present are not usually pathogens and have little opportunity to grow. Each mechanically-ventilated patient must be supplied with an adequately decontaminated set of connecting tubing but it need not necessarily be sterile. Tubing washed and dried in a washer with a heat disinfection cycle is usually acceptable. The required frequency for changing the connecting tubing of a respiratory ventilator is the subject of some controversy with recommendations varying from 6 to 48 hours. Although 24 hours is considered the optimum, studies indicate little additional risk

**Table 18 Contamination levels of patient expiratory tubing at end of session**

| Method of treatment | No. of samples | No. of samples showing | | |
|---|---|---|---|---|
| | | Moderate/heavy growth | No growth | Gram-negative bacilli |
| Autoclaved at end of previous session | 11 | 0 | 4 (36%) | 0 |
| Chemical disinfection with glutaraldehyde | 8 | 0 | 3 (37%) | 1 (12%) |
| Not treated | 5 | 5 (100%) | 0 | 5 (100%) |

if changed at 48 hours or even 72 hours[28]. The use of a filter placed near to the patient's mouth can protect the tubing and keep it dry for longer periods[40]. The internal circuitry of the machine is usually protected by filters, but where this is not the case the machine will require changing every few days and decontaminating after each use.

Re-processing non-disposable equipment to an adequate standard is often difficult and when carried out in individual wards or units, standards tend to vary. Sufficient space and suitable equipment are rarely available. Optimal conditions can best be provided in a well-planned, carefully controlled, specialist equipment cleaning section in the Sterile Services Department, where trained staff clean and autoclave special equipment and where adequate space can be made available. Additional stocks may be required to allow for the extra processing, packaging and transport time. Savings can, however, be made in some major items once a reliable standard of decontamination and servicing is achieved. A central pool of available equipment can reduce the amount of stored unused equipment on wards and should ensure that a smaller proportion of available equipment is out of service at any one time.

## Endoscopes

Despite the considerable increase in use of flexible fibreoptic endoscopes, reports of transmission of infection are uncommon. *Ps. aeruginosa* and other Gram-negative bacilli have been transferred from the endoscope to other patients and clinical infections have occurred, particularly after endoscopic retrograde cholangio-pancreaticography (ERCP). *Salmonella* spread has also been associated with gastroscopy, but there is little evidence of transmission of mycobacteria or hepatitis B virus and, as yet, none of HIV[48]. Most of these episodes of infection have been associated with inadequate cleaning and disinfection. The problems of endoscopes and cleaning are: narrow channels i.e. suction, air, water, which are difficult to clean, some components are heat-labile, and residual fluid in the endoscope, water bottle, or even in the washing machine may allow the growth of *Ps. aeruginosa* and other opportunistic Gram-negative bacilli after overnight storage. Decontamination of the water bottle is particularly important, also the water compartment of an automatic machine. The rapid turnover of patients, e.g. every 15 minutes, leaves little time for effective cleaning and disinfection. Automatic machines and fully immersible endoscopes are useful aids to rapid and

**Table 19 Disinfection of endoscopes using an automated system**

| Agent | No. of tests | Mean log reduction |
|---|---|---|
| 2% Glutaraldehyde | 49 | 3.59 |
| 70% Ethanol | 17 | 3.81 |
| QAC disinfectant cleaner (Dettox) | 37 | 3.43 |
| Neutral detergent | 17 | 2.50 |

effective processing and few residual organisms remain (Table 19)[49, 50]. Exposure to 2% glutaraldehyde for 1–2 minutes should kill most vegetative bacteria and inactivate most viruses[51], including HIV. A longer exposure, e.g. 4 minutes is recommended as a routine and in association with good cleaning should further reduce the risk of transfer of HBV; 70% alcohol is an alternative for disinfection of the channels, but may damage the endoscope if immersed. However, wiping the insertion tube after thorough washing will leave few residual organisms. Effective cleaning with a detergent will remove most contamination and a quaternary ammonium compound (QAC) such as 'Dettox' is effective but will not necessarily inactivate viruses. Mycobacteria are more resistant to glutaraldehyde and bronchoscopes should be exposed for at least 30 minutes. If associated with thorough preliminary cleaning, this should prevent transfer of mycobacteria. However, 60 minutes exposure to glutaraldehyde should be considered following use on a known infected case.

# Chapter 9

# Sterilization

Sterilization is usually described as the complete destruction or removal of all micro-organisms. In practice, defining the required standard is more difficult. The size of the load and the speed at which effective penetration of the sterilizing agent occurs must also be considered. It may be unreasonable to expect rapid penetration into a well-packed container full of sand or to kill $10^{10}$ bacterial spores in serum. Nevertheless, if the definition is to be fulfilled any organisms likely to be present should be killed and there should be a reasonable safety margin. Killing $10^6$ bacterial spores of a defined resistance to the process is a commonly accepted standard. Autoclaving at high temperatures will usually meet the required standard with a very large safety margin.

Problems occur with heat-labile equipment where the probable pre-sterilization count may have to be considered. A process such as low temperature steam and formaldehyde which can be expected to kill $10^4$ spores may be acceptable as a sterilization process for cleaned endoscopes where spore counts are expected to be well below this figure. This method would be more reliable than the use of a fluid chemical disinfectant because of superior penetration, although the disinfectant may have a similar potential for killing spores. It may be preferable to describe such methods as decontamination adequate for a defined purpose, rather than sterilization[52].

Other methods with little sporicidal action such as pasteurization or a short immersion in glutaraldehyde may cause less damage to sensitive instruments and be more rapid and convenient. The use of such methods may allow more patients to be treated in each session without substantially increasing the risk of infection, since there is a high probability that all the organisms present on a washed instrument will be killed. The probability of the process rendering the item sterile is, however, less than the probability using a conventional sterilizing technique such as autoclaving, and the process should not be described as sterilization.

Methods of sterilizing include dry and moist heat, filtration, irradiation, ethylene oxide gas, low temperature steam with formaldehyde (LTS/F) and chemicals with a sporicidal action, e.g. formaldehyde, glutaraldehyde and buffered hypochlorites. The preferred method of sterilizing, which should be used whenever possible, is steam at increased pressure (autoclaving), but alternative methods are required for heat and pressure-sensitive items.

## Autoclaving

An autoclave is a pressure vessel supplied with steam which is held at a constant pressure for a set period of time. The temperature of pure steam is related to its

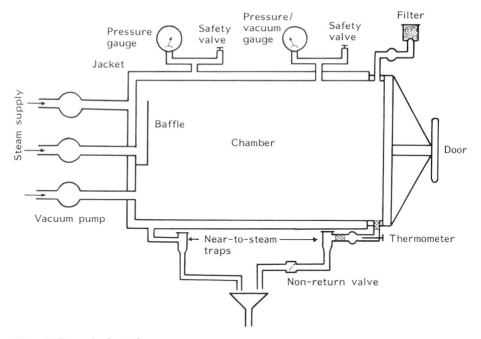

**Figure 20** Porous load autoclave

pressure. Autoclaves range from little more than a pressure cooker to a highly complex piece of equipment costing many thousands of pounds. A sophisticated autoclave is required to ensure safety, reliability and to reduce the damage caused by heat and pressure (Figure 20). Accurate adjustment of pressure, time and temperature will provide an acceptable sterilizing or holding time, which is the time the temperature is maintained after the most difficult part of the load to penetrate has reached the required temperature (Table 20). Less complicated sterilization equipment such as a modified pressure cooker may be an acceptable alternative where personal responsibility for ensuring the time, temperature and pressure relationships can be taken by a professional individual, e.g. dentist or chiropodist operating outside hospital premises. These machines are capable of sterilizing but do not have automatic control and monitoring equipment to the level of HTM10 (to be published) required in hospitals. They are, however, preferable to the other alternatives used, e.g. chemical disinfection, ultraviolet irradiation or hot water, etc. which do not sterilize. Steam penetrates well, but is only effective when relatively free of air. With porous loads or complex equipment, vacuum extraction

**Table 20 Relationship between autoclave pressure and temperature**

| Pressure (lb per sq in) | Temperature (°C) | Sterilizing time (min) |
|---|---|---|
| 15 | 121 | 15 |
| 20 | 126 | 10 |
| 30 | 134 | 3 |

may be necessary to ensure air is adequately removed. The effect of small amounts of residual air remains controversial. The Bowie-Dick test for removal of air should be carried out daily on all high vacuum (porous load) autoclaves. In this test a cross of autoclave tape on a sheet of paper is placed in the centre of a standard pack of towels; uniform intensity of the darker stripes throughout the entire length of both strips of tape indicates adequate air removal. Towel packs could be variable in thickness and moisture content because of variations in wear, frequency of laundering and variations in airing time. A more reproducible test cube (the Lantor Cube) which simulates the towel pack is now produced and widely used as an alternative. The test is quite sensitive since the residual air tends to accumulate in the centre of the pack. Spores are not routinely used for monitoring steam sterilization in the UK since their heat sensitivity may be variable and microbiological tests are less reliable than physical methods of monitoring.

The monitoring of sterilization of bottled fluids is more complex and requires that a thermocouple is placed in a typical container in the coolest part of the autoclave. A door lock mechanism which prevents the autoclave being opened before bottles have cooled to 80°C is also required, otherwise bottles may explode when removed due to sudden changes in pressure.

The pressure vessel of the autoclave is a huge energy store and any sudden or uncontrolled release of that pressure can be highly dangerous. These factors have led to rigorous control and testing of equipment by the Department of Health and Social Security (HTM10). Autoclaving requires expensive capital equipment and should preferably be carried out under careful control by trained staff in a centralized department. Sterilized goods exposed to the air do not remain sterile, and proper arrangements for packaging, storage and handling of sterilized items are an essential part of the process. However, for unwrapped instruments for immediate use a simple process of exposure to steam is usually acceptable, providing the autoclave is well maintained.

## Dry heat

Dry heat penetrates less well and is less effective than moist heat. Higher temperatures and longer time periods, e.g. 160°C for 60 minutes, 180°C for 30 minutes, are required for sterilization as well as a longer heating-up time. This method is used infrequently, for although metal instruments and heat-resistant glass will often withstand these temperatures, heat distortion can occur, lubricants tend to dry and many other materials become brittle or scorched. The total heating-up, holding and cooling time may be several hours. Sterilizing ovens should have a time lock on the door so that items cannot be added or removed during the cycle, and a fan to distribute the heat evenly.

## Low temperature steam and formaldehyde (LTS/F)[53, 54]

A combination of steam under reduced pressure to give a temperature between 70 and 80°C (e.g. 73°C with a range of +5°C or −2°C) and formaldehyde gas can achieve sterilization under specified conditions, but does not give the same margins of safety as a conventional autoclave. However, this process may cause considerably less damage to heat-sensitive materials, although some of the advantages may be lost in longer cycle times. Low temperature steam alone (73 + 5 − 2°C) for 10 minutes is an effective means of disinfection and is particularly useful for respiratory equipment likely to be damaged at higher temperatures. Spores, usually *Bacillus stearothermophilus,* must be used for monitoring LTS/F processes since it is partly a chemical method, although indicators may be satisfactory as a supplement to spores if rigorously controlled. Reproducibility of spore preparations is a problem which is under investigation, but at present care is required since some test pieces contain few viable spores.

# Ethylene oxide gas sterilization[55, 56]

Ethylene oxide sterilization is usually confined to industry or large hospitals. The gas is toxic and very careful control of temperature, humidity, pressure and gas concentration is essential. Ventilation of the environment in which the ethylene oxide sterilizer is situated must also be controlled. Toxic vapours can be absorbed into some materials and long aeration times can be speeded up by forced-draught ventilation. There has recently been some concern particularly in the USA that ethylene oxide may be carcinogenic, but in practice the risks appear to be small if safety conditions are fulfilled. This equipment is usually used for sterilization of manufactured goods, such as plastics, in which the expected microbial contamination is low. Microbiological controls are usually used, e.g. aluminium strips carrying at least $10^6$ *Bacillus subtilis* var. *niger* spores, often in association with chemical indicators.

## Irradiation

Gamma irradiation is used industrially to sterilize many disposable plastics after packing. The cost, size of sterilizing equipment and necessary control measures make this an uneconomical method for use in hospitals. The range of items that can be irradiated without causing unacceptable changes is limited, and many items will not withstand repeated irradiation without damage. Plastics often become more brittle. Care is necessary if different methods of processing are used on the same equipment, e.g. irradiation followed by ethylene oxide or glutaraldehyde.

## Filtration

Fluids and gases can be sterilized by passing them through a filter with a fine enough pore size to retain microbes. This method is very difficult to control and it is difficult to determine whether microbes have leaked around the sides of the holder or escaped through small holes in the filter. The pressure required to force fluids through the filters can change their composition and there is always some loss of volume. While an efficient filter may remove bacteria from solutions it will not necessarily remove preformed toxins, and contaminated fluids which are to be administered to people cannot necessarily be rendered safe by filtration. This process is not accepted as sterilization by some workers and alternative methods are preferred when possible.

# Sterilization by chemical solutions

When it is not possible to use heat or the other methods already described, fluids may have to be used for sterilizing, but only if more efficient alternative methods are not possible. Any fluid that can kill a sufficient number and range of bacterial spores can be described as a sterilizing agent or 'sterilant', and includes strong mineral acids and a number of other chemicals. Sterilization by this method is theoretically possible, but difficult to achieve reliably in practice. Grease, coagulated protein or even a layer of air can easily prevent any fluid coming into contact with the microbes contaminating the surface. The bacterial spore is a resting phase with a hard shell and does not readily take up fluid from its surroundings. The chemical has to dissolve, break down or penetrate that shell to kill the organisms. Unfortunately, it is often more resistant to such chemical attack than the surface to be sterilized. Highly concentrated chemicals or prolonged exposure is often required, which can result in damage to the surface to be sterilized. Time can also be an important factor. The results obtained with the United States AOAC (Association of Official Analytical Chemists) test indicates that the required exposure time for sterilizing with 2% glutaraldehyde is 10 hours, although in the UK 3 hours is acceptable[57]. Formaldehyde vapour is also sporicidal but it is unpleasant, toxic, does not penetrate well and has to be neutralized after use. However, prolonged exposure (e.g. overnight in a safety cabinet) will kill spores.

Glutaraldehyde is commonly used for heat-sensitive equipment. It is expensive, often unpleasant to handle, allergenic, and the residual glutaraldehyde is potentially toxic. Treated equipment requires thorough rinsing. Grease, protein and other soil must be removed before immersion. Residual air in lumen of needles, corrugated tubing or fine channels tends to prevent adequate contact. The treated instrument is wet after rinsing, and microbial recontamination is always possible. Glutaraldehyde solutions may be either acid or alkaline. Alkaline glutaraldehydes tend to be the more active, but less stable than acid preparations. Their efficacy declines after activation and can usually be used for only 14 days. More stable alkaline glutaraldehydes remaining active for up to 1 month are available, but some caution is required. If the solution is activated and unused it will remain active for that period, but if repeatedly used it may be partially neutralized or considerably diluted. Continuous use for more than 2 weeks is probably the outside limit, and solutions should be discarded if they become visibly cloudy at any time. Ideally, a previously unused solution should be used each time, but the cost would be prohibitive. The number of uses allowable for a solution must depend on circumstances and an indication of the strength of a solution is required if repeatedly used.

Many new glutaraldehydes have appeared on the market and vary in activity and corrosiveness[57]. It should not be presumed that an instrument which is not damaged by one brand of glutaraldehyde will be safe in another. Items exposed to glutaraldehyde for under 3 hours should be regarded as disinfected, not sterilized.

Hypochlorites, particularly if buffered to pH 7.6, are more rapidly active against spores than glutaraldehydes and are capable of killing them in minutes, but unfortunately hypochlorites are readily inactivated, corrode metals and attack some plastics and rubber. Iodine and iodophors belong to the same group and although sporicidal are usually too slow in activity to be reliably used routinely as sterilizing agents.

Sodium dichloroisocyanurate (NaDCC) can be used as an alternative chlorine release agent and is considered by some workers to be less corrosive. Chlorine releasing agents are stable in tablet form with a shelf life of years and are particularly useful when occasional use only is required. These agents are preferable to liquid formulations but tend to be more expensive (see also Chapter 10).

# Disinfection

Disinfection involves the destruction of microbes but not necessarily bacterial spores. Ideally, all vegetative microbes should be killed, but a reduction in the number of pathogens to a level that is unlikely to cause infection is usually acceptable.

Products and procedures described in trade and other literature may not adequately decontaminate items when the surface has been contaminated with highly resistant or unusual organisms, or if excessive numbers are present. Residual organisms present after disinfection may still be an infection risk to the unusually susceptible patient (see Chapter 2). When choosing a disinfectant for a specific hospital use it may be necessary to know the numbers and types of organisms likely to be present and the susceptibility of the patients involved. Products and procedures as described by manufacturers may therefore not always be suitable for hospital use, and disinfectants chosen for one purpose may not be equally effective if used for another.

## Heat disinfection[58]

Heat is less selective, more penetrative and easier to control than most liquid chemical disinfectants. Heat is, therefore, the preferred method of disinfection. Vegetative organisms will usually be killed when exposed to moist heat at 65°C or above. The length of time the item needs to be exposed will depend on the temperature. Timing of the disinfection process should not start until the coldest part of the load has reached the required temperature. If this is unknown or cannot be measured, additional time must be allowed for all items to reach the required temperature.

The following temperatures can be used as guidelines:

(a) 65°C for 10 minutes.
(b) 70°C for 2 minutes.
(c) 80°C for 1 minute.
(d) 90°C for 1 second.

These are times based on the killing of *Strep. faecalis* which is more resistant to heat than most vegetative organisms and viruses. It may therefore be possible to disinfect heat-sensitive items at lower temperatures for longer times. Damage caused by heat will increase as the temperature is raised and with the duration of time it is held at that temperature. Disinfection temperatures and times agreed for heat-labile equipment should not be increased arbitrarily by the operator, since a safety margin is usually built into the recommended temperature. Since steam penetrates more readily than hot water and hot water more readily than dry heat, the more penetrative methods will be faster and should be chosen in preference.

## Chemical disinfectants[59]

Chemicals are usually applied as fluids but gases, e.g. formaldehyde vapour, are more penetrative. There are a number of conditions determining the effectiveness of chemical solutions:

1. Satisfactory contact – it may be difficult to ensure that the fluid comes into contact with all contaminated surfaces. Grease film or protein coating may prevent contact between the contaminated surface and the disinfectant.
2. Neutralization – a wide range of substances including hard water, soaps, detergents and certain chemicals, which include some plastics used in the manufacture of cleaning equipment, e.g. lavatory brushes, may neutralize the disinfectant.
3. Concentration of the disinfectant – while it is obvious that if the disinfectant is too weak it may not be effective, it is not so well appreciated that phenolics, alcohols and disinfectants that contain wetting agents and stabilizers may be less efficient if the concentration is too high. Disinfectant dilutions should always be accurately measured.
4. Stability – not all disinfectants are stable, particularly when diluted, and may deteriorate with storage. Disinfectant dilutions should preferably be freshly prepared for use, but if issued at use dilution should be marked with an expiry date.
5. Speed of action – a disinfectant may act slowly but be chosen for other advantages. Alcohol is rapid in action but penetrates poorly. Hypochlorites are also rapid but at high concentrations are corrosive. They are very cheap and at low concentrations can be effective, are relatively non-toxic, but are readily neutralized. Clear, soluble phenolics have a wide spectrum of activity, are not readily neutralized, act reasonably fast and are inexpensive. Glutaraldehyde is expensive, but is an effective sporicidal agent and less likely to damage expensive equipment than hypochlorites or clear soluble phenolics.
6. Range of action – disinfectants are not usually equally effective against the whole range of microbes likely to be present. Cetrimide, hexachlorophane and, to some extent, chlorhexidine are all less active against Gram-negative bacilli than Gram-positive cocci. Many disinfectants have poor activity against fungi or specific viruses. Hypochlorites (and glutaraldehyde) are more active against HBV than most other disinfectants and are preferred where there is a hepatitis B or HIV risk.

Cost is a relevant factor when choosing disinfectants. Those designed for special purposes, e.g. 'Savlon' and chlorhexidine for skin disinfection, may be both unsuitable and too expensive for use as a general environmental disinfectant. To be used safely on human tissue a disinfectant would have to be non-toxic, non-allergic, non-corrosive and have a neutral pH. These properties are expensive to achieve and are usually obtained at the expense of other desirable properties, e.g. range of activity.

**Disinfectants commonly used in hospitals**

Aldehydes and hypochlorites are active against most viruses; 70% alcohol is active against enveloped, but less so against non-enveloped, viruses; phenols, iodophors and QACs are variable in their antiviral activity. 'Slow' viruses are resistant to aldehydes. These and some of their properties are shown in Table 21.

*Clear soluble phenolics (e.g. 'Clearsol', 'Stericol', 'Hycolin')*
These are widely used for disinfection of the inanimate environment and are active against a wide range of bacteria including tubercle bacilli, but not against most bacterial spores or some viruses. They are toxic and to some extent corrosive, and are unsuitable for use on living tissues or any item brought into contact with tissues unless thoroughly rinsed. Phenolics should not be used for the disinfection of food preparation or storage surfaces due to the strong smell and possibility of tainting food. Damage may be caused to surfaces on prolonged or repeated contact, or if too concentrated solutions are used. Clear soluble phenolics are relatively cheap, usually stable at use dilutions and are not readily neutralized by organic materials. Compatible detergents may be included in the formulation to aid cleaning, but detergents or other cleaning products should not be added by the user. Clear soluble phenolics are usually used at a concentration of 1–2%.

*Hypochlorites*
Commercially available hypochlorite (bleach), e.g. Chloros, Domestos, Sterite, Parazone, etc. contain a nominal 100 000 parts per million (ppm) available chlorine but the concentration may be very much higher or lower than the nominal concentration depending on the age of the solution. Hypochlorite tablets are more stable and have a long shelf life. If diluted according to the manufacturer's recommendation they will give accurate concentrations but they are more expensive. Sodium dichloroisocyanurate (NaDCC) can be used as an alternative to hypochlorite solution and is usually diluted to give the same level of available chlorine but is regarded as more active and less corrosive[60].
  Bleach diluted 1 in 10 to give 10 000 ppm available chlorine is used to disinfect blood spillage likely to contain HBV or HIV, but at this strength it is toxic, corrosive and likely to bleach fabrics. Diluted 1 in 100 (1000 ppm) hypochlorite can be used for environmental decontamination but may still corrode metals and bleach fabrics. Milton is a stabilized hypochlorite solution containing 10 000 ppm available chlorine diluted 1 in 80 to give a concentration of 125 ppm available chlorine. It is used to disinfect infant's feeding equipment and other items to be used in contact with food. Hypochlorite at concentrations of between 1 and 5 ppm available chlorine may also be used to disinfect swimming baths and drinking water. Hypochlorite is also used in high concentrations for cleaning toilets and sanitary ware, but if mixed with acid descalers will react violently and may produce toxic chlorine gas.

*Iodine and iodophors*
Iodine is also a halogen and has many similar properties to hypochlorites. It is less commonly used for environmental disinfection, but is more often used as a skin disinfectant. Its main disadvantage is that it may stain fabrics brown, or react with the starch in fabrics to produce a blue stain. Iodophors consist of iodine and a

solubilizer, and are relatively non-toxic. They can be washed from fabrics more readily than iodine. The depth of colour is related to activity and this may be used as an indicator although this relationship is not entirely reliable. Iodophors are more expensive than hypochlorites and allergy is less likely than with iodine.

### Chlorhexidine

Chlorhexidine is a sophisticated and relatively expensive disinfectant of low toxicity formulated primarily for clinical use. It is most active against Gram-positive cocci, e.g. *Staph. aureus,* and is less active against Gram-negative bacilli; it has low activity against tubercle bacilli and is not significantly sporicidal. Virucidal activity is generally poor. Chlorhexidine may be inactivated in the presence of soap. This product should not be used to disinfect inanimate objects unless its lack of toxicity or compatibility with human tissue is of major importance.

**Table 21 Properties of disinfectants**

|  | Activity against | | | | Inactivated by | | Corrosive action |
|---|---|---|---|---|---|---|---|
|  | GPC | GNB | Spores | TB | Protein | Soap |  |
| Phenolics |  |  |  |  |  |  |  |
| Sudol | ++ | ++ | − | + | ± | − | + |
| Izal | ++ | ++ | − | − | ± | − | − |
| Soluble phenolics* | ++ | ++ | − | + | ± | − | ± to + |
| Pine | ± | ± | − | − | ++ | − | − |
| Dettol | ++ | + | − | − | ++ | − | − |
| Chlorine compounds | ++ | ++ | ++ | + | ++ | − | ++ or ±† |
| Iodophors | ++ | ++ | + (slow) | + | + | − | − |
| QAC‡ | ++ | ± | − | − | ++ | ++ | − |
| Tego | ++ | ± | − | − | + | ++ | − |
| Chlorhexidine | ++ | + | − | − | + | ++ | − |
| 70% alcohol | ++ | ++ | − | + | ++ | − | − |
| Formaldehyde | ++ | ++ | ++ (slow) | ++ (slow) | + | − | + (slow) |
| Glutaraldehyde | ++ | ++ | ++ (slow) | ++ (slow) | ± | − | ± |

*Stericol, Clearsol, Hycolin. ‡Quaternary ammonium compounds.
†Buffered solutions.
GPC Gram-positive cocci.
GNB Gram-negative bacilli.
++    High.
+    Moderate.
±    Low.
−    Nil.

### 'Savlon'

This contains chlorhexidine and cetrimide. It has an inherent detergent property which makes it useful for cleaning dirty wounds. Both constituents are inactivated by soap and it is less active than an equivalent dilution of chlorhexidine alone, but properties and use are similar. It is not recommended for environmental disinfection.

## Alcohol

Ethyl alcohol 70% or isopropyl alcohol 60% is rapidly active against most vegetative bacteria and enveloped viruses, but has little or no activity against bacterial spores. Since alcohol acts rapidly but penetrates poorly its main use is for the rapid disinfection of physically clean surfaces, e.g. dressing trolley tops, hands or injection sites. Its other advantage is that it evaporates rapidly and leaves the surface dry and can be used for some equipment which may be damaged by other agents. Ethyl alcohol is very inflammable and care should be taken in storage. Isopropyl alcohol is rather less inflammable.

# Chapter 11

# Cleaning

Cleaning is necessary to maintain the appearance, structure and efficient function of a hospital and its contents. Cleaning may also be required to control the microbial population and to prevent transfer of infection. Cleaning alone may be sufficient to do this, but it is also required as a preliminary to satisfactory disinfection or sterilization. However, disinfection or sterilization of some contaminated items may occasionally be necessary prior to cleaning to allow safer handling, but this may not be reliable.

Cleaning is a process intended to remove any substance ('soil') that is not part of the structure or designed to assist the function of the item being cleaned. This objective may be modified by practicalities or cost. Cleaning should be achieved without shortening the life or interfering with the function of the item being cleaned. Any item after cleaning should have fewer organisms present on its surface and be a lower infection risk. Contaminated water-soiled mops or wipes may add to the number of organisms present. The source of 'soil' including microbiological contamination may be from particles deposited from the air or transferred by contact with people or other objects. Cleaning to the standards in hospitals requires specialized training and may also require specialized equipment, methods and materials.

## Appearance

A clean appearance is important to patients and staff. Failure to meet expected standards can seriously reduce confidence in the ability of the hospital to provide adequate treatment. 'Soil' may also mask identification marks, warnings or instructions on equipment.

## Structure and function

'Soil' may corrode, abrade or react chemically with a surface. It may also block channels, interfere with valves or the flow of liquids, gases or electric current, or encourage the presence of insects or other pests. Moisture alone may cause rusting or corrosion, providing conditions in which microbes can grow, or which can interfere with electrical circuits. Drying is therefore an essential part of the overall cleaning process. Residual 'soil' may prevent the penetration of heat or chemicals required for disinfection or sterilization.

# Cleaning procedures

Cleaning should remove and not redistribute 'soil' or microbes. After 'soil' has been removed it should be disposed of safely, and the method of disposal always requires careful consideration in hospitals. Cleaning should not increase the number of microbes in the surrounding environment and any redispersal of pathogens should be kept to a minimum. If a technique which disperses organisms into the air cannot be avoided it should not be carried out in the immediate vicinity of exposed wounds or other susceptible sites; a sufficient time, at least 15 minutes, should preferably be allowed for dispersed organisms to settle.

Some areas of the environment, e.g. drains, toilets and sink outlets, are naturally heavily contaminated with Gram-negative bacteria, and cleaning will only have a very temporary influence on their numbers. Although these areas must be kept clean it is often more sensible to regard them as contaminated and to take any necessary precautions rather than to adopt expensive but ineffective measures and then ignore the risk. However, risks of infection from drains, toilets and sinks are generally small (see Chapter 8).

# Methods of cleaning

Two basic methods of cleaning are used, dry and wet. If a dry method is used, dispersal of bacteria-carrying particles into the air is the main infection risk. The organisms mainly involved will be Gram-positive cocci and diphtheroids from the skin, but *Staph. aureus* is the main common hazard. Anaerobic spore-bearing bacilli such as *Cl. welchii* or *Cl. tetani* may be present in small numbers. These organisms will only cause infection if inoculated into deep, oxygen-deficient tissues and their presence in small numbers in the environment is not a cause for concern. Dry methods rely on mechanical action to loosen and remove larger objects and particulate soil, but do not remove stains and are unsuitable for wet or greasy surfaces.

### Sweeping

Brooms tend to redisperse bacteria-laden particles into the air even when used with care and may increase the airborne count by as much as tenfold (see Figure 17). Dispersed dust will then resettle. Sweeping is, therefore, potentially hazardous and inefficient, and should be avoided in patient treatment or food preparation areas.

### Dry mops

Mops which are specially treated or manufactured to attract and retain dust particles cause smaller increase in airborne counts and remove more dust from surfaces than brooms[61] (Table 22). Tests suggest that dry mops require washing or reprocessing after about 2 days' use; their dust-holding properties may be extended to 4 or 5 days if the head is vacuumed after each use. The method of use is important if dispersal is to be avoided; the head of the mop should be kept flat and in close contact with the floor and not tilted or lifted at the end of each stroke. Mops of this type with a disposable head are available, but are more expensive.

**Table 22 Changes in airborne bacterial counts associated with different methods of cleaning floors**

| Method used | Change in bacterial count |
|---|---|
| 1. Sweeping with broom | 700% increase |
| 2. Vacuum cleaning | 20% decrease |
| 3. Dust-attracting floor mop | 30% increase |
| 4. Wet scrubbing machine | 3% increase |

The effect may vary with the make of equipment and method of use.

## Vacuum cleaning

Vacuum cleaning with a well-designed vacuum cleaner should not increase airborne counts, providing the exhausted air is passed through a bacteria-retaining filter (Table 22). The expelled air from the cleaners should be diffused and directed so that it does not blow dust from uncleaned surfaces back into the air.

## Surface cleaning

Dry dusting, particularly high dusting, may shower dust onto the patient. Damp dusting is preferable although dry dusting can be carried out with a vacuum head or a dust-retaining mop. If there is a danger of dispersing dust, all open wounds should be kept covered until at least 15 minutes after dusting has ceased.

## Wet cleaning

Solvents or water-containing detergents may be used to resuspend or dissolve adherent soil. Dispersal of microbes into the air is less likely during wet cleaning than dry cleaning. However, cleaning solutions soon become contaminated and bacteria may grow in them. Any splashes or aerosols produced by wet cleaning may be contaminated and should be kept to a minimum. Used cleaning solutions should be disposed of promptly and safely. When cleaning with a single bucket the bacteria removed from the surface are transferred to the bucket; the water should be changed frequently or a two bucket system should be used. It is usually necessary, particularly in operating theatres, to rinse after cleaning as detergents or soap will become concentrated on the surface when the fluid dries and there is a build-up of a detergent film. This will increase the rate of soil accumulation, interfere with the antistatic properties of theatre floors and may attack some floor finishes. The film may also interfere with subsequent floor treatments by preventing bonding to the surface. Soap film is also a common cause of slippery floors. Moist surfaces encourage bacterial growth and should be regarded as potentially contaminated. After cleaning, preparation surfaces in food and clinical areas should not be used until completely dry. Routine cleaning should be carried out as part of an agreed policy with detailed agreed schedules. Hospital policy should be given preference where it conflicts with the manufacturer's instructions, but it is always a good idea to read the instructions first and clarify any discrepancies.

# Outline policy for good cleaning practice

1. Prepare a fresh cleaning solution, accurately diluted for each task. Make up only the quantity required in a clean, dry container. Freshly drawn tap water is usually suitable, but very hard water will precipitate soaps and neutralize some disinfectants. Hot water cleans better than cold, but at temperatures above 65°C it coagulates protein, e.g. milk and blood, and stains will then be more difficult to remove.
2. Apply the cleaning solution evenly to all of the surfaces. If a brush, mop or wipe is used it should be clean and preferably dry before use.
3. Do not put more fluid than necessary onto a surface. This avoids waste, seepage into cracks, shrinkage of materials and difficulties in subsequent removal.
4. Change the solution frequently to prevent a build-up of soil or microbes in the solution which would recontaminate the surface.
5. Allow sufficient time for cleaning solutions to penetrate the soil on the surface, but also remember that strong acid and alkaline cleaning agents can damage surfaces if left in contact for too long.
6. Rinse off cleaning solutions when practical.
7. Dispose of used cleaning solution promptly in the dirty utility area. Do not discard into wash-basins or clinical sinks.
8. Remove any fluid trapped in channels or elsewhere and dry the cleaned surface as thoroughly as possible.
9. Remove cleaning equipment from clinical treatment or food preparation area as soon as possible; it should then be cleaned, dried and stored in the designated place. If the equipment is faulty it should be reported promptly to a supervisor.
10. Wash hands before carrying out any other duties.

Hospital cleaning is a specialized task which requires trained staff who will keep to the detailed schedules produced by the domestic manager in consultation with other disciplines, e.g. the manager of the area and the microbiologist or a member of the Infection Control Staff. Alternative methods or materials should not be used unless authorized. Cleaning products should not be mixed unless known to be compatible; soaps or detergents will often reduce the effectiveness of disinfectants, and some products may react in a dangerous manner, e.g. soap may neutralize quaternary ammonium compounds and acid cleaners will react with hypochlorites (bleach) to produce a poisonous gas, chlorine. Surface deterioration is often caused by inappropriate cleaning. Not all commonly used cleaning techniques in hospitals have been introduced as properly planned, co-ordinated, adequately researched policies, and it is reasonable to check methods which do not appear to be soundly based. It is part of the job of Infection Control Staff to liaise with other disciplines in evaluation of the need for changes in existing procedures and policies related to infection risk.

# Cleaning of isolation cubicles and other special risk areas

Specialized techniques which are not justified for other areas may be required for rooms occupied by infected or highly susceptible patients, e.g. isolation units, operating theatres and intensive care units. Detailed schedules for cleaning these areas should be produced in consultation with nursing and medical staff, the microbiologist or other Infection Control Staff, and the domestic manager. Techniques vary with circumstances. Disinfection is not usually necessary but firm decisions should be made as to whether or not it is required.

The following objectives should be considered when formulating the policy:

1. Microbial contamination from the infected patient should be contained within that environment.
2. The patient should be protected from any further infection.
3. Anyone with access to that environment should be aware of the measures required to prevent any further spread of infection.
4. After use by an infected patient the environment should be made safe for any future use, and it should be apparent that this has been done.

The following outline draft of a cleaning policy for an isolation cubicle includes some of the main aspects to be considered:

1. The sister in charge of the ward should notify the domestic supervisor as soon as possible that special cleaning is required. The domestic supervisor should then ensure that:
   (a) The correct procedure is known and understood by the domestic staff responsible and that suitable equipment and materials are available;
   (b) The domestic staff are sufficiently aware of any risks to themselves or others and are adequately protected, e.g. if the patient has open tuberculosis, tuberculin-positive staff are used;
   (c) Cubicles are cleaned in the right order, e.g. the cubicles used for the isolation of highly susceptible patients should be cleaned first, and cleaning staff should not re-enter that cubicle until all cleaning of cubicles for infected patients has been completed and suitable measures to prevent transfer are taken.
2. Equipment should be reserved for use in the specified area only, and clearly marked for that purpose; it must be stored in this area or in a clearly defined place outside it. Where this is not possible, equipment must be adequately decontaminated immediately after each use. Mechanical cleaning equipment should be avoided if possible in isolation rooms for infected patients, but if used a separate brush or head should be reserved for that area and should be decontaminated, preferably by autoclaving before re-use elsewhere. The outside of the machine should be wiped after use with a clear soluble phenolic, or, if not appropriate, 70% alcohol. Scrubbing machines with tanks are particularly difficult to decontaminate and their use should be avoided in these circumstances. Disposable wipes which can be discarded inside the isolation cubicle prevents their accidental re-use in other areas.

Cleaning equipment should be kept to a minimum. The following will usually be sufficient:

A plastic bag for the disposal of refuse.
A bowl for damp dusting, preferably kept in the cubicle.
Disinfectant solution if required.
A mop and bucket designated for use in that area only.
Disposable paper wipes.

## Procedure

1. Collect all the equipment required for cleaning.
2. Enter the cubicle, wash hands, put on disposable apron and gloves.
3. Pick up any large items of rubbish and discard in plastic bag, also empty into the bag. Sweeping is not acceptable and a vacuum cleaner is usually impracticable unless a separate machine is available for each cubicle.
4. Clean floor with a damp mop.
5. Make up a solution of disinfectant (if required) in a bowl. Use disposable wipes moistened in the solution and discard after each use. Clean structural surfaces first, including door handles. Clean furnishings, starting with the locker and finishing with the waste bin and sink. Discard remaining solution in bucket, wipe the bowl and return to the storage area in the cubicle.
6. Remove gloves and plastic apron, if single use, and discard into plastic bag; seal bag, wash and dry hands.
7. Leave the cubicle; take with you the sealed rubbish bag and any item of equipment not stored in the cubicle. Buckets should be emptied, dried and returned to storage area. Occasionally it is specified that the cleaning water is disposed of inside the cubicle, although this is undesirable. This means that potentially contaminated fluids are tipped into a hand-basin or toilet, possibly splashing the recently cleaned environment. If this is necessary, reserve some cleaning solution in the bowl to re-clean the sink and splashes. If cleaning water is removed from the cubicle it should be taken immediately to the dirty utility room, discarded, the bucket cleaned and the hands washed.

When an infected patient is removed from an isolation cubicle a notice, e.g. 'Do not use', should be put on the door. The notice should only be removed by a senior nurse after checking that all necessary decontamination measures have been taken to ensure that the cubicle is safe to occupy.

## Contract cleaning

All staff employed in catering or patient treatment areas should have an appropriate knowledge of food hygiene and infection control procedures relevant to their area of work. Where a requirement exists for health service staff to have medical checks or to be immunized against specific infections, e.g. tetanus, rubella or tuberculosis, this should also apply to contractor's staff. These requirements should be included in contracts. The cost of training and medical services supplied to contractors by Health Authorities should be considered in costings.

Materials, methods and equipment used by contractors should conform to existing hospital policy, e.g. disinfectants used in compliance with policy, the restriction of transfer of cleaning equipment from one area to another and hot water spray extractors used only according to an approved code of practice. Supervision of the contract to ensure safety and compliance is important but those expected to provide the monitoring service, e.g. Infection Control Staff, should be consulted first. Effective monitoring can require considerable time, specialized skills and laboratory resources. Microbiologists, Infection Control Nurses and other staff who may be expected to carry out this task may not have the resources available, and the importance of this task should be considered in relationship to their existing priorities. Some flexibility should exist within contracts to allow for additional requirements during outbreaks.

# Chapter 12

# Cleaning, disinfection or sterilization?

## Choice of method

It is sometimes difficult to make a choice between these methods; each is usually progressively more expensive and more likely to damage the structure or function of the item and to keep it out of commission for a longer time. There is little sense in an elaborate process of sterilization if the organisms present are unlikely to cause infection or will re-appear before the equipment is next used.

To obtain a completely sterile environment would be prohibitive in cost and would be impractical as well as unnecessary. Even if achieved, it could not be maintained if people were present in the environment. There is little point, even in disinfection, if a reduction in bacterial numbers is not associated with a reduction in infection risk, or the reduction cannot be maintained. Disinfecting a toilet seat once a week could affect the risk of infection for the next user, but not for the subsequent users over that week. A more logical approach is to identify individuals who are likely to contaminate the seat with specific pathogens and always disinfect after use by them. The following notes may assist in making a logical choice.

## Sterilization

Sterilization is required in situations where small numbers of surviving organisms may cause infection because of enhanced opportunity to reach a susceptible site, or where the organisms are particularly resistant to other forms of treatment, or are exceptionally virulent. Sterilization may also be required if surviving organisms can multiply on the item and are likely to reach an infective dose on subsequent storage.

The main requirements for sterilization are as follows:

1. Surgical instruments or dressings in contact with exposed tissue; items or substances introduced into an otherwise sterile area of the body, e.g. infusion fluids; topical applications to broken skin if the agents are capable of supporting growth of potential pathogens or allowing them to survive.
2. Where contamination with potentially pathogenic spores in significant numbers is likely, e.g. *Clostridium tetani, Cl. welchii, Cl. botulinum, Bacillus anthracis* or equipment contaminated with highly virulent life-threatening microbes not normally found in the environment, e.g. the viruses associated with Marburg disease, Lassa and Ebola fevers.

3. In situations where disinfection would normally be acceptable but the items are required for an environment where exceptionally susceptible patients are being treated, e.g. leukaemics or transplant patients. This is a less certain indication and disinfection or thorough cleaning is usually adequate.
4. Occasionally to preserve substances, usually fluids, which can be broken down by bacterial action.

## Disinfection

Disinfection is required to reduce the numbers of pathogenic microbes to a safe level, where there is a definite risk that they will reach a susceptible site, and if sterilization is not required or is impractical.

The main requirements are as follows:

1. Cleaning contaminated spillage, e.g. blood, pus, urine, vomit or faeces, from known infected patients.
2. Decontamination of an environment occupied by a person with a known transmissible disease where the next occupant will be at risk for infection; cleaning alone will usually be sufficient.
3. The treatment of items likely to be brought into direct or prolonged contact with a patient, e.g. bed linen, if contamination is likely from its previous use. Disinfection is usually part of the hospital laundering process. Bedpans and urinals will require disinfection when used by infected patients, but cleaning and drying alone after use by non-infected patients may be acceptable.
4. The routine cleaning of high risk areas, e.g. operating theatres and intensive care units, but cleaning alone should usually be sufficient.

## Cleaning

This is the removal of accumulated deposits by washing with a cleaning solution, or by the dry abrasion of the surface, e.g. dry mopping. This will reduce microbial contamination by the physical removal of organisms and substances which will support their growth or attach them to the surface.

Cleaning is usually adequate for any item that does not come into prolonged close contact with susceptible individuals and where there is no specific reason to suspect contamination by spillage of infectious material.

# Chapter 13

# Laundering

Hospital linen and clothing should be laundered between patients, or if it becomes visibly soiled, or at least weekly. The laundry process should remove evidence of previous use, including organisms, even though the risk of surviving organisms causing infection in a subsequent user is small. Laundry items are not sterile, since small numbers of microbes will be deposited on them from the air and during handling.

Although no standards are available and routine microbiological testing is unnecessary, the following guidelines may be helpful if there is a problem with the process. The average mean microbial count from the surface of used hospital linen is between 10 and 20 organisms/sq cm when sampled with contact plates (25 sq cm). These consist predominantly of Gram-negative bacilli (about 50%), skin organisms and aerobic spore-bearing bacilli. After washing and drying and before despatch, the majority of organisms are likely to be coagulase-negative Gram-positive cocci in small numbers. The number of organisms should be reduced to approximately 1/sq cm or less on sampling with a contact plate[62]. The presence of larger numbers of Gram-negative bacilli after washing suggests that recontamination has occurred during the later stages of the process, e.g. from presses or recirculated water. It may also indicate inadequate drying. High counts of *Staph. aureus* or *Strep. faecalis* are suggestive of inadequate heat disinfection. Laundering is not a sterilization process and cannot be expected to kill bacterial spores, although in practice they are not usually present in large numbers.

**Handling of hospital linen** (see general notes on handling contaminated hospital waste, Chapter 15)

Used linen should be removed from the patient or bed with care. Unnecessary agitation of fabrics can markedly increase the number of bacteria in the air. It is possible, though not very likely, that a single fibre shed from the linen of the patient with a staphylococcal infection may contain sufficient bacteria to initiate an infection if it settles on a susceptible wound. However, these particles are quite large and will resettle rapidly. It is preferable that susceptible wounds are not exposed within 15 minutes of bed-making, although this is not always possible. Used linen should not be counted or sorted in the patient environment, and even when enclosed in a bag and properly closed it should not be handled roughly, dropped or kicked, as this may force contaminated aerosols or particles into the ward air.

Failure to remove foreign objects, particularly if metal or sharp, e.g. needles or scissors, from used linen can cause extensive and very expensive damage to laundry machinery or infect sorting personnel. This is particularly important for categories of linen enclosed in water-soluble bags which will be placed in machines unopened. If this problem could be eliminated and sorting avoided, categorizing would be unnecessary and all linen (apart from heat-labile) could be treated in the same way.

Any used linen may be contaminated with potential pathogens. The risk of these organisms infecting a healthy person is small if reasonable care is taken even when items are visibly fouled, provided they are handled with care. The most important measure to prevent transfer of infection is good handwashing procedure. Hands must always be washed after handling used linen; all used linen should, however, be sealed as soon as possible in a bag which is impervious to microbes. If water is able to penetrate the surface of the bag, it is probable it will also enable microbes to pass through the bag. Laundry bags should, therefore, not be stored in wet places and must be protected during transport.

The category of linen inside a laundry container should be clearly indicated on the outside. The following colour coding is taken from the recently published DHSS guidelines HC(87)30:

'Used' but not 'infected': a white or off-white bag.
'Infected': a red bag, or with red as a prominent feature on a white or off-white background.
'Heat-labile': blue or white bag with a blue stripe.


## Disinfection and categories of laundry

Wherever possible all used hospital laundry should be heat disinfected in the washing process and although there are occasional failures, disinfection is usually completed in the drying and pressing stages (Figure 21). However, hazards of

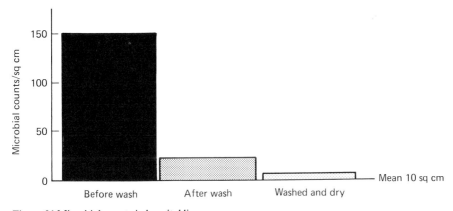

**Figure 21** Microbial counts in hospital linen

transfer of infection following a low temperature wash are probably small and a requirement for disinfection by heat in the washing stage may be considered to be unnecessary for some routine laundering in the future.

**Temperature requirements**

All hospital linen capable of withstanding the required temperature should be heat disinfected during a wash cycle. The temperature of that cycle should reach a minimum of 65°C (150°F) for not less than 10 minutes or preferably 71°C (160°F) for not less than 3 minutes (Figure 22). These temperatures must be reached and maintained in the coolest part of the load. A sufficient pre-heating time must be

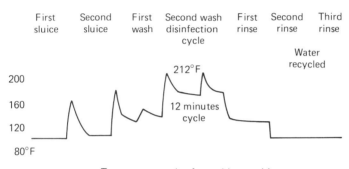

Temperature cycle of a washing machine

**Figure 22** Temperature profile of a laundry process

allowed for the required temperature to be reached. The time required will vary with the machine and the load, but at least 5 minutes will usually be required. Most vegetative bacteria and viruses, including HIV, are heat-sensitive and should be readily killed at 71°C for 3 minutes. Although the minimal temperature required to kill HBV is unknown, the combined washing and heat processing should render the linen safe. Removal of blood secretions is the essential part of the decontamination process.

# Categories of linen

The previous DHSS guidelines HM(71)49, recommended that linen should be divided into two main categories:

1. Foul or 'infected': consisting of items visibly soiled with human excretions or secretions, or known to have been in contact with a patient suffering from a range of specified infections.
2. Soiled: consisting of all other used linen.

Foul or 'infected' items were to be contained in a water-soluble bag and placed directly into the washing machine without sorting. This has caused problems. Considerable sorting was required at ward level, the cost of soluble bags was often high, since in some laundries the majority of items to be washed were from geriatric units and classified as 'foul' or 'infected'. Machines were damaged by sharp items accidently included in unsorted loads. Heat-sensitive fabrics were not removed and therefore damaged by the heat disinfection cycle. For these reasons some managers considered it necessary to sort foul or 'infected' linen. This meant that linen that had been in contact with patients with specific human infections, possibly transmissible by this route, was inadvertently handled since it was not separately identified. Although the risk of transmission was small it was felt to be unacceptable. The new recommendations HC(87)30 included a change of classification to:

1. Used (soiled and fouled): all used linen not covered by other named categories. However, if it is operatively convenient to divide used linen into soiled and fouled, there is no reason why this should not be done, but it is not a requirement. It is difficult to justify the cost of water-soluble bags, separate machines or separate handling areas for fouled linen.
2. The 'infected' category contains linen from patients with or suspected of suffering from enteric fever, other salmonella infections, dysentery, tuberculosis, hepatitis B, HIV infection, some notifiable diseases and other infections in hazard group 3 (ACDP, 1984)[63] or other infections specified by the Infection Control Officer. Although it is recognized that linen which is not fouled or blood-stained from these patients is probably of low risk and that any linen may be contaminated from unknown carriers, it would seem rational to separate this group, unless sorting can be eliminated and the contents transferred to a washing machine without handling. However, linen from most notifiable diseases is not hazardous and could be treated in the usual manner. Linen potentially contaminated with organisms in hazard group 4 should be steam sterilized on site before laundering. Linen in the 'infected' category should be sealed in a water-soluble bag at the point of use and then placed in an outer bag. The outer bag should be impervious and colour coded in accordance with SIB(10)20. This bag should be washed at the same time as the contents. The water-soluble bag should be placed unopened in a machine known to have an efficient heat disinfection cycle.
3. The heat-labile category includes fabrics likely to be damaged by the temperature required for thermal disinfection. Where these would otherwise have been categorized as 'infected' they will require chemical disinfection. Hypochlorites containing 150 ppm available chlorine added to the penultimate rinse is suggested, but there is a need to develop and test other chemicals for this purpose.

## Risk to laundry workers

Fouled linen, unless from patients with known or suspected gastrointestinal infection, is likely to be contaminated with the same organisms as other used linen though they may be present in greater numbers. These organisms usually consist of the normal faecal flora and are unlikely to cause infections in healthy laundry workers, providing care is taken. *Staphylococcus aureus* (including MRSA) are unlikely to represent a hazard to laundry staff.

Protective clothing should be provided for those handling used linen prior to the disinfection stage. This should include good quality rubber gloves, overalls, a plastic apron and, where required, waterproof boots. The laundry worker should not leave the laundry in potentially contaminated clothing and preferably it should not be possible to enter or leave the area where used linen is handled without passing through a room provided with at least a wash hand-basin. The provision of shower and changing facilities is also recommended. It is essential that workers handling used linen before the disinfection stage are taught the importance of washing their hands before leaving the work area as well as the benefit of wearing the protective clothing provided.

Staff should have a normal chest X-ray on employment and should be tuberculin positive, or show evidence of a successful BCG vaccination. Immunization against poliomyelitis and tetanus should be offered Typhoid vaccination is of uncertain value, and is rarely advised. The risk of transfer of hepatitis B to laundry workers is remote provided hygienic precautions are taken; immunization is not recommended at the present time, but should be considered in future immunization programmes. The Occupational Health Department will advise on immunization requirements.

## Tunnel or continuous washers

Continuous or batch continuous washers are increasingly being used in hospitals. Work carried out by the Infection Research Laboratory has shown that they can disinfect to an acceptable standard if they are properly commissioned and maintained. However, recontamination of the finished product may occur and is more likely to occur if recycled water is used. Organisms tend to grow overnight while the machine is not in operation, and it is usually recommended that the machine is run until empty and then heat disinfected before restarting. This adds considerably to running costs. Microbiological tests for commissioning and checking in the case of outbreaks or disputes have been published[62] and these would help to detect major failures or substantial recontamination. Routine microbiological monitoring is not recommended.

## Domestic washing machines in small units

Domestic type washing machines are increasingly used in small units or because it is felt that the hospital laundry damages personal clothing, such as knitted items. These machines may be acceptable where those using the clothing are reasonably healthy, but not for infected or immunocompromised patients. It is particularly important that the clothing is thoroughly dried after washing. If there is any doubt a microbiological check of the finished product may be useful. If the total count on a contact plate is not more than 1 organism/sq cm, the process is probably acceptable. It is advised that a laundry process with a heat disinfection cycle is used during outbreaks of infection. As the potential hazard is dependent on the type of infection, advice should be obtained from Infection Control Staff.

# The use of commercial laundries

Where hospital laundering is subcontracted to an outside laundry, hospital policy relating to disinfection should be followed and steps should be taken to ensure that the proposed process will adequately disinfect. Measures considered necessary to protect hospital staff when handling used linen should also apply to non-hospital staff handling the same type of material and this should include appropriate immunization.

Chapter 14

# Catering

The hospitalized patient is more susceptible to food-borne infection and more likely to suffer serious consequence from such infection than healthy members of the community. It is difficult to compare the risk of food-borne infection related in hospitals with the risk from food prepared elsewhere. Not only will a high proportion of hospital patients be more susceptible but the chance of food-borne infection being diagnosed and recorded is very much higher in the hospitalized patient. The tendency to centralize food preparation in hospitals also means that a single lapse in food hygiene can put large numbers at risk. In our own district, 60 000 meals are prepared each week and in the near future these will all be prepared in a single production unit. The risk of acquiring food poisoning from eating a meal in the large hospital where our laboratory is situated is approximately 1 in 40 million. However, since food is prepared for a particularly susceptible population, the highest possible general standards must be maintained.

The removal of Crown Exemption in the UK has raised problems unlikely to occur in other sectors of the catering industry. There is sometimes an expectation amongst Environmental Health Officers that higher standards than those prescribed by law should operate in hospitals. In commercial catering establishments, the cost of work requested by an Environmental Health Officer will come from profits, and even if it results in the business closing, there will usually be an alternative available to the customer. The net result should be an overall reduction in infection risk and a potential improvement in the health of the group involved. However, in the hospital there is no alternative source of food and the hospital may need to be closed while improvements are made. The cost will have to be diverted from other health care needs, including possible measures intended to reduce more serious infection risks in other areas where there is not a mandatory requirement. The need to comply with food hygiene regulations intended to reduce risk and improve health could in the hospital situation increase infection risk and cause an overall deterioration in the health of patients. Good communication between the manager responsible for diverting the resources, the Environmental Health Officer and the Infection Control Officer is essential if a balance is to be maintained. It is essential that this legislation does not operate to the overall disadvantage of the sick patient.

Detailed policy which concentrates on the correct purchasing, handling, processing and distribution of food is more important then environmental conditions, although on casual inspection a poor state of decoration and repair and superficial soiling is easier to detect. To maintain appropriate standards continuous training and supervision is more important than occasional inspections. A genuine risk assessment of the procedures is probably more effective than an over-rigorous enforcement of possibly outdated legislation. The ending of Crown Immunity does not in any way reduce the responsibility of the hospital Infection Control Officer to assess overall risk of infection and see that available resources are allocated in accordance with the degree of risk.

Food poisoning may occur if relatively large numbers of specific organisms or preformed microbial toxins are consumed. This usually occurs because the organisms have been allowed to multiply unchecked in food.

*Salmonella* spp. are the commonest cause of outbreaks of food poisoning (80%). The infective dose is about 10 000 organisms for a healthy person. *Salmonella* spp., *Staphylococcus aureus* and *Clostridium welchii* may be present in humans and animals without causing infection and are common contaminants of raw meat, fish and poultry. The following control measures are recommended:

1. Good separation of naturally contaminated food from food already cooked or likely to be eaten without cooking.
2. Adequate cooking to destroy causative organisms and some of the more heat-labile toxins.
3. Storage at a temperature likely to prevent the multiplication of micro-organisms.
4. High standards of catering and personal hygiene promoted by adequate training and enforced by constant supervision.

Difficulties can arise when food preparation is used as occupational therapy for those not fully capable of understanding the basis of good food hygiene. The food cooked in such exercises should not be shared with other groups.

## Adequate cooking

Destruction of micro-organisms depends on exposure of the food to an adequate temperature for a defined time. Most cooking procedures should destroy vegetative bacteria if the process is well controlled. Heat penetrates dense masses slowly and minimal temperatures may be found in the coldest part of the load, e.g. the centre of the thickest part of a joint of meat, or a container of mashed potato or milk pudding. Few cooking processes can guarantee to kill heat-resistant spores. A balance must be maintained between adequate cooking and ruining good food by excessive heat. Measurement of the temperature of food during cooking or at the end of the cooking period is rarely carried out and the more frequent use of a suitable thermometer with an appropriate probe for sampling the internal temperature of food masses is recommended (Figure 23). Any surface which has reached 65°C and is maintained at that temperature for 10 minutes or has reached 80°C for even a few seconds is unlikely to be heavily contaminated with vegetative organisms. The presence of unaltered haemoglobin, in the fluid or meat, suggests that temperatures above 60°C have not been reached. In one test, the internal temperature of a joint of beef described by the chef as 'well done' did not exceed 42°C during the process. Rare (undercooked) beef is preferred by many people and rarely causes harm but it can be responsible for outbreaks of infection and should not be given to hospital patients. Undercooked poultry or pork is never acceptable. The use of carefully defined menus, which include the maximum size of joints and minimum cooking temperatures and times, is strongly recommended. Policies for

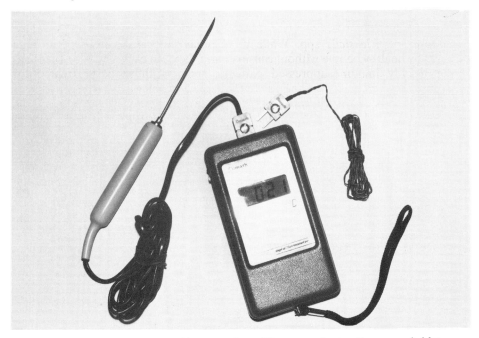

**Figure 23** Small digital thermometer with meat probe and thermocouple wire. Recommended for checking heat processes and heating equipment

the re-use of food prepared for other purposes and the length of time which food, once prepared, can be stored before discarding should be included.

Cooking times are usually based on the process starting at room temperature, and inadequate defrosting of frozen products can lead to substantial and hazardous undercooking. Once adequately cooked, the temperature of the food should be retained at 63°C or above until eaten. Reheating of cooked food should be avoided except as part of a properly planned chilled meal service. Where this is unavoidable it should be cooled rapidly and stored at 4°C or below until required. Large joints of meat and bulk foods may cool very slowly; the centre may remain at bacterial growth temperature for long periods, even if refrigerated. Using small joints and spreading mince, etc. out on trays will facilitate rapid cooling. Cooked foods capable of supporting bacterial growth, e.g. soups and gravies, which will be stored and reheated, should not remain out of the refrigerator for more than 2 hours. No part of the food should be at a temperature of above 6°C and below 60°C for more than 4 hours. Food kept at these temperatures for longer periods is not necessarily inedible or unsafe, but with good management these guidelines can be achieved in hospital practice. It must also be appreciated that when reheating food in stock or sauces the temperature of that stock or sauce is not necessarily an indication of the temperature of the food within it. Catering staff should use temperature measuring equipment regularly and particularly when adopting new procedures.

## Salad vegetables and fruit

Salad vegetables served uncooked should always be examined carefully and well washed under running water before being served. They are frequently heavily contaminated with a wide range of Gram-negative bacilli including *E. coli, Ps. aeruginosa* and *Klebsiella* spp. While these organisms can be ingested in large numbers by healthy people without causing harm they can cause invasive infections in the heavily immunosuppressed patients, such as those being treated for leukaemia, and it may be necessary to serve only cooked food to such patients (see Table 23). The skin of fruit may also be contaminated and should be washed and dried. It is preferable to remove the skin immediately before the fruit is eaten by the very susceptible patient.

**Table 23 Bacterial isolates from food**

| Types of food | No. of samples | No. of samples containing viable bacteria |
|---|---|---|
| Food served hot | 70 | 28 (40%) |
| Cold foods: salads, cooked meats, etc. | 61 | 52 (85%) |

Organisms isolated included *E. coli* (33), *Enterobacter* and *Klebsiella* spp. (25), and *Ps. aeruginosa* (8). Thirty-five samples of cold food had counts in excess of 5000 organisms/g.

## Segregation of cooked and uncooked food

Raw meat and poultry, fresh fish and raw vegetables should all be assumed to be contaminated with potential food poisoning organisms. Separate preparation areas, each with their own equipment and staff, should ideally be provided. Although fish can be prepared in the meat bay, there is a risk of transferring the distinctive odour and taste of the raw fish to the meat. Plastic aprons are usually worn for preparing these foods. These aprons should be removed and the hands thoroughly washed and dried by staff before handling any food that will be eaten without further heat treatment. If implements or other materials which have been in contact with raw meat, fish, poultry or raw vegetables have to be used for other purposes, they must be properly washed and thoroughly dried before re-use.

## Storage

Any food which contains moisture should be stored at temperatures below 6°C. This will prevent the multiplication of most bacteria, but will not kill existing bacteria. There are certain obvious exceptions, such as raw fruit and vegetables, which may be stored for short periods without refrigeration. Although most food poisoning organisms are unlikely to grow below 6°C, bacterial enzymes which cause food spoilage may remain active. Deep-freezing at −18°C will inhibit most enzymes but will not kill bacteria.

## Food preparation surfaces, crockery and cutlery

Detailed schedules defining methods, material and frequency of cleaning for each item should be produced and displayed in each department. The schedules should define who is responsible for carrying out each task and supervision should be based on the written schedules. While it is probable that fluctuation in demand or absence of staff will make it difficult to maintain schedules on occasions, clearly indicated priorities will ensure that essential work is carried out.

Food preparation surfaces should be clean and dry before use. The commonest cause of heavily contaminated food preparation surfaces is recent cleaning with a contaminated cloth and failure to allow sufficient time for the surface to dry thoroughly. While it is recommended that stainless steel or other impermeable surfaces are used this is less important than good cleaning and thorough drying, preferably using a disposable paper wipe or clean dry cloth. If a good technique is used, disinfection is rarely needed and is never a substitute for good technique.

**Table 24 Bacterial counts from washed plates**

| Method | No. sampled | Counts of 10 or more per contact plate (25 sq cm) |
| --- | --- | --- |
| Hand-washed | 108 | 68 (63%) |
| Machine-washed | 72 | 5  (7%) |

Crockery and cutlery washed in a machine with a final rinse temperature of 80°C or above, and allowed to dry before use, should be microbiologically safe. This is more efficient than washing by hand even with a detergent/disinfectant solution (Table 24). Washing by hand should preferably be carried out in a double sink with a final rinse in clean hot water. Visibly moist crockery or cutlery should not be used but disinfection may not be required except after use by infected patients, or during outbreaks. Disinfectants are never required if adequate temperatures are reached during the washing and rinsing processes[64].

## Handwashing

It is necessary to instruct food handlers specifically when, where and how to wash their hands. Recent work has shown that even well trained nurses can miss vital areas such as tips of fingers or thumbs when not properly instructed (see Figure 15). A wash-basin reserved exclusively for handwashing, with a designated person responsible for ensuring that soap and paper towels are always available, should be provided at each work bay. It is difficult to persuade caterers (or any other staff) to walk more then a few feet to wash their hands. Poorly sited wash-basins are not used. Washing with soap and water is generally adequate and disinfectants are unnecessary unless recommended by the Infection Control Officer during outbreaks. All food handlers should receive some basic training in food and personal hygiene.

## General comments

Equipment which is intended to keep food at a controlled temperature, either hot or cold, should be checked regularly and wherever practical a clearly visible thermometer should be incorporated as part of the equipment. A daily inspection by a supervisor or manager to ensure that equipment is operating at the right temperature and that storage policy, e.g. separation, is understood and carried out is recommended.

Complaints of undercooking or of keeping hot food below the required temperature should be investigated thoroughly. Failure to maintain standards on one occasion could result in a disastrous outbreak.

Heated food trolleys are intended to keep hot food warm and not to heat food. Hot food must, therefore, be at a temperature of 63°C or above when placed in the trolley. A period of approximately 30 minutes should be allowed for the trolleys to reach the required temperature before use and they must be kept on until food service is completed. The ability of the trolley to maintain food at the appropriate temperature can deteriorate and should be checked at regular intervals (monthly).

## Investigation of outbreaks[65]

It is essential to plan in advance the action to be taken in the event of an outbreak. A Major Outbreaks Committee should be in existence (see Chapter 4) and the roles and responsibilities of its members clearly defined[3]. To ensure that any outbreak is recognized as soon as possible, proper documentation of all cases occurring in either patients or staff is required. The completed documents should be forwarded as soon as possible to one responsible person, preferably the Infection Control Officer. Enquiries should then be made to ensure these are genuine cases and to establish whether they meet the pre-defined criterion for informing the Major Outbreaks Committee. Information on type of symptoms, time of onset and dietary history over the previous 48 hours is of value. The dietary history of uninfected controls may also be helpful. Wherever possible arrangements should be made to send specimens to the laboratory before staff are sent off duty.

The source of staphylococcal food poisoning is often an infected lesion or rash in a food handler. *Salmonella* usually originates from poultry inadequately defrosted before cooking or due to poor personal hygiene in a carrier. Staff should always be questioned about recent infections or attacks of sickness or diarrhoea in themselves or their families. Large outbreaks which persist and do not all appear to have originated from a single food item or on a specific day may suggest contaminated equipment or a persistent carrier. Since multiple infections are unlikely unless the bacteria have had an opportunity to multiply after contamination, it is highly probable that food was kept at the wrong temperature for too long and this should always be investigated. A slowly spreading infection with the number of cases building up over some days is rarely food poisoning. A small number of scattered patients recently admitted may reflect infection contracted outside the hospital, even if all of the same type, if that strain is common in the community. If all infected patients have eaten the same food it is highly probable that this is the cause, but because of variations in susceptibility and the amount consumed it would be unlikely that all those consuming the contaminated food would be infected.

## Faecal screening

Outbreaks are rarely due to faecal carriers and even if routine tests are made this does not guarantee that all carriers will be identified or that epidemics are less likely. Screening gives a false sense of security. Hygiene standards should be high enough to ensure that food is not contaminated with faecal organisms. Screening policies are often irrational; carriers may excrete only very rarely, perhaps once a year. If staff were screened before employment, annually or even every 6 months, they may well become infected the next day, or be missed. Screening for typhoid carriers may be a justifiable precaution in countries, or in staff from countries, where typhoid is common. Carriers are difficult to cure and any sudden introduction of a screening programme may well mean the loss of staff who, despite their carriage, have worked safely and well for many years.

Much larger numbers of enteric pathogens may be excreted immediately after an infection than in a chronic carrier even though symptoms have disappeared, and it is essential that catering staff are trained and actively encouraged to report any incident of diarrhoea or vomiting in themselves or their families. They are, however, unlikely to be co-operative if temporary absence from the normal duties leads to loss of pay.

## Pre-cooked chilled foods

There has been a rapid expansion in the use of pre-cooked chilled meals in hospitals. In this system food is cooked, packed, rapidly chilled and stored refrigerated for up to 5 days before being portioned and distributed. The food is then reheated (regenerated) in purpose-built equipment immediately prior to consumption. The advantage of this system is that it enables the work load of kitchens to be spread over a longer period, reducing peak demands at meal times. It should also provide a greater variety of menu, but does lead to increasing centralization. The centralization and increased storage time involved could be expected to increase the risk of food-borne infection. In practice the degree of control and monitoring built into pre-cooked chill systems, usually absent from traditional catering systems, adequately compensates for the increased risk. There has as yet been no outbreak of food-borne infection associated with cook-chilled foods in hospital. Careful examination of working systems has, however, shown that with some practices there can be an unacceptable increase in the level of organisms present[66].

New systems require detailed planning well in advance of construction. A flow chart of the proposed system should be prepared from the arrival of the food on site to the final point of consumption. Each stage should be examined for potential infection risks. The correct work flow patterns and the permissible time and temperature range for each type of food passing through an area should be agreed. Monitoring systems to ensure that the accepted parameters are not exceeded should also be set up and the relevant documentation prepared. A clear chain of command and responsibility should also be established. Any readings taken, e.g. temperatures, must be reviewed by a manager who will accept responsibility for taking action or not doing so. Changes may have to be made in the light of operational experience, but systems should be in place before operations commence. The DHSS guidelines on pre-cooked chilled foods[67] should be used as a basis for drawing up operational systems. The basic requirements of these guidelines is that following cooking, food should be reduced to a temperature of 3°C within 90 minutes and then stored at a temperature of 3°C for not longer than 5 days, including the day of preparation and the day of consumption.

If during storage the temperature of the food rises to 5°C it must be consumed within 12 hours and if it rises to 10°C it should be discarded. These guidelines do, however, include substantial safety margins and over-rigorous interpretation can erode potential cost savings without reducing infection risks and can adversely affect the acceptability of the food served. Consultation with the local Environmental Health Officer at an early stage is advised but it is important to differentiate between advice given as a legal requirement and personal preference of the Officer giving it. Requirements should be clearly backed by law or should be a clearly demonstrable risk that can be backed with microbiological evidence or case histories. The Environmental Officer of Health should be asked to differentiate and provide evidence if necessary. Where it is decided that departure from the guidelines is necessary the reason for doing so should be recorded and the process should be monitored microbiologically until it is considered safe. The records should be kept permanently. Any problem should be referred to the Infection Control Officer. The microbiological quality of the food should be at an acceptable level prior to regeneration and regeneration temperatures should not be relied on to render it safe. Not all foods are equally suitable for this process, though this may depend on the method of regeneration. Some gravies and sauces may separate and skinned and sliced meat can dry out. Dishes with a high moisture content, such as casseroles, may be most suitable but it cannot be assumed that traditional dishes can necessarily be prepared by this method. Regular monitoring of the temperature of the regenerated food is required. Monitoring should not always be from the same point or the same trolley, since failure of a single plate can occur unnoticed. Each trolley should be marked so that tests are carried out in rotation and all points are tested over a given period.

Extensive microbiological testing may be necessary at the initial stages to ensure that all systems are working consistently and to a reliable standard. However, when the physical parameters necessary to ensure this have been established, microbiological monitoring can be considerably reduced. Recording thermometers on all refrigeration plants are recommended.

Some organisms may survive or even multiply at the temperatures used for storing chilled food, e.g. *Listeria* spp. The risk from such organisms can, however, be readily exaggerated. They tend to occur in a limited range of products, including goat's cheese and commercially prepared salads. These products are often kept at low temperatures for very long periods and are unlikely to be part of a hospital diet. However, a careful watch is required for potential pathogens that may grow at low temperatures, since there are increasing reports of food poisoning by these organisms.

# Chapter 15

# Waste disposal

Domestic and clinical waste are likely to contain moisture and protein which will allow organisms to multiply. Since Gram-negative bacilli are commonly present and will grow more readily than other organisms, these will usually predominate regardless of the source of the waste material. All waste should therefore be regarded as heavily contaminated and handled with care.

The general public consider certain items of hospital waste as offensive, e.g. incontinence pads, used dressings and, regardless of their source or level of microbial contamination, presume they are an unacceptable infection risk. There is no evidence that infection has been acquired from clinical waste, apart possibly from needles. There is also a small amount of waste likely to be contaminated with specific human pathogens not normally found as environmental contaminants and needing special handling. However, if this category is too wide it is likely to cause unnecessary expense and down-grade the risk and care taken with the more genuine high risk material. The DHSS document HN(82)22 gives guidance on the safe disposal of clinical waste and on the colour coding of waste containers. Since the removal of Crown Immunity, hospitals do have a legal responsibility for the safe disposal of hazardous waste. This is not necessarily discharged by handing it over to a contractor without checking that the contractor is competent and responsible. There is also a responsibility to ensure that resources are not wasted on excessive measures which are out of proportion to actual risk. Close co-operation with the Health and Safety Executive is required to reach a balanced approach. It has become increasingly difficult to obtain quotations for the disposal of some categories of hospital waste and hospitals may be forced into providing on-site incineration or secure transport to Health Authority-operated incinerators. This is unnecessarily expensive and not warranted by the actual risk to personnel.

## Categories of waste

It is always possible that some waste will be wrongly classified or that one individual will regard items as offensive which are acceptable to others. It is, therefore, preferable that where practical, hospital waste is incinerated.

### Domestic waste

The majority of waste generated within the hospital is no greater risk than waste generated in a house or other public buildings. It is illogical that waste acceptable as domestic waste from these sources should not be acceptable from a hospital.

Domestic waste includes all material not mentioned in subsequent categories. Domestic waste should be discarded into *black plastic bags*, the tops of which should be securely closed when full. It is important that bags are not overfilled so that they can be properly sealed.

### Clinical waste

This category should include all material predictably contaminated with microbes known to cause specific human infections and not normally found in substantial numbers in the environment, e.g. material contaminated with blood, excreta or secretions from cases of hepatitis B, HIV infection, tuberculosis, salmonellosis, enteric fevers or other infections specified by the microbiologist.

Clinical waste should be sealed in *yellow plastic bags* and disposed of by incineration. Storage in a secure area while awaiting collection is required.

Used dressings, incontinence pads and wipes used to clean up incontinent patients are not a specific infection risk. These items would, however, undoubtedly be considered offensive in bulk if recognizable. If incinerated on site there is probably no need to separate them. Incineration is preferable, but they can be disposed of by landfill if special arrangements are made to ensure they are not likely to be left uncovered or accessible to the general public. Where there is sufficient of these items to represent a problem, they can either be treated separately and put into *yellow plastic bags with a black stripe* or, if more convenient and economical, included as clinical waste. These items are discarded as domestic waste in the community and there is no microbiological reason why this practice should not continue.

### Sharps

All needles and sharp instruments for disposal should be discarded into a sharps box to DHSS specification TSS/S/330.015 (see also HN(80)22 and (HEI)11/76 and 74/78). These should not at any time be kept where they are readily accessible to children, e.g. in hospital corridors, and should not be placed on a wet surface. Temporary storage must be secure. Sharps containers should not be handled more than necessary since penetration of the container can occur. It may be necessary for the hospital to make arrangements for the safe disposal of clinical waste and sharps used by community services.

### Human tissue

Where there is a need to dispose of identifiable human tissue it should be immediately enclosed in a *yellow plastic bag* and transported to an operating incinerator under the supervision of a responsible person and placed directly into the incinerator. If an operating incinerator is not immediately available it should be stored in a mortuary until incineration can be arranged. If it is necessary to transport limbs or other tissues outside of the hospital for disposal, the yellow plastic bag should be placed inside a rigid locked container labelled 'Waste requiring special disposal, please contact Mr . . . Tel no . . .'. These are contingency arrangements to prevent offence if the vehicle is involved in an accident.

**Laboratory waste**

All cultures and patient specimens for discard and any items that have been in contact with the culture or specimen should be made microbiologically safe before leaving the laboratory usually by autoclaving. Incineration of combustible materials is an acceptable alternative and if transport is necessary should be treated as clinical waste.

Most other waste from the laboratory that has not been in contact with laboratory waste or specimens can be regarded as domestic waste.

**Other categories of waste requiring special treatment** (see HN(82)22)

1. Cytotoxic drugs and other specified pharmaceuticals.
2. Certain chemical waste including corrosive, toxic and inflammable materials.
3. Radioactive material.

**Waste which may require separation**

Broken glass, aerosol canisters, food waste, scrap metals and used photographic materials for silver recovery fall into this group.

# Storage

Storage sites should be properly planned, sited to avoid offence, secured against access by unauthorized personnel, cats, dogs, mice, birds and other pests, and should be protected from the weather. The area should be cleaned at regular intervals. Poorly maintained refuse areas attract vermin which may open bags and distribute the contaminated contents over the surrounding environment. While there is little evidence of any major infections having been spread in this manner, it is clearly undesirable. Refuse storage areas can also attract children in search of syringes, etc. as toys, itinerant dealers in search of saleable scrap, and mentally handicapped patients who are unaware of potential hazards. Security is therefore of some importance.

# Collection

Since discarded waste is a nidus for multiplying microbes, it should be removed from the patient environment at regular intervals. Collection should be approximately twice daily and not less than daily from wards. It is preferable to collect hazardous materials, e.g human tissue, sputum pots, etc. separately to prevent mixing with other refuse.

# Disposal of faeces, urine, waste water, etc.

Large numbers of the general population outside hospital become infected with enteric pathogens. They may carry pathogens on their skin or excrete them in their urine or faeces without symptoms. These organisms are often *Salmonella* spp., occasionally including *S. typhi*. Even when these carriers are identified, public authorities do not require that urine, faeces or waste water is disinfected before discharge into the sewage system; to do so would be totally impracticable. *Salmonella* spp. causing food poisoning are probably the commonest enteric pathogens and a high proportion of people who contract this disease do not seek medical treatment and are rarely hospitalized. The number of pathogenic microbes from this and almost every other common infection discharged into the sewage system from outside the hospitals will therefore be greatly in excess of the numbers discharged into that same system from within hospitals. It would, therefore, seem illogical to attempt to kill the smaller number of pathogens before discharge from hospital material while doing nothing about the much larger number from outside the hospital. This would be expensive, extremely difficult, would worry the patients concerned, and would have a negligible effect on the infection risk involved from contact with untreated sewage. There is indeed a possibility that to put vast additional amounts of disinfectant into the sewage system could kill the microbes that we rely on to make it safe.

There are a few exceptions where unusally severe infections, such as Lassa and other haemorrhagic fevers, are so potentially hazardous that they are treated in special units where sewage is treated before discharge. However, there is an obvious risk in transferring infection when handling material from patients with enteric infections and the bedpans or urinals should be heat disinfected, preferably in a correctly designed bedpan washer with a heat disinfection cycle[58]. Alternatively, the entire contents with the pan or urinal can be disposed of in a macerator which should have a good door seal and lock and be properly maintained so that it does not produce contaminated aerosols.

Transporting used bedpans from patients with enteric infections from one ward to another should be avoided if possible and the contents should be disposed of promptly. Storage may enable *Salmonella* etc., to multiply thus increasing the risk of transferring an infective dose. If chemical disinfection is required when a washer with a disinfection cycle or a macerator is not available, the pan or urinal should be emptied, rinsed and then disinfected with 1% Stericol or a similar phenolic for 20–30 minutes, then rinsed thoroughly and dried. If a soak tank is used the disinfectant may rapidly become neutralized, or resistant bacteria may emerge. The disinfectant solution will then contaminate rather than disinfect subsequent items. When disposing of urine, faeces or other contaminated fluids, such as used cleaning water, it should be remembered that it is likely to be highly contaminated, and disposal should be into a sluice, sink or lavatory. If a wash-basin, kitchen or clinical sink is used, contamination may be transferred to hands, food or equipment. Covering faeces in a bedpan with a chemical disinfectant is of limited value as sufficient penetration to reduce substantially the number of pathogens present is unlikely, and the gross excess of protein present may rapidly inactivate the disinfectant. The reduction in risk is minimal and may give a false sense of security. Leaving the pan full of disinfectant and faeces in a sluice room for 30–60 minutes increases the risk of spillage and dissemination of infection.

# Chapter 16

# Special units

## Hospital sterile services department

The function of a hospital sterile services department (HSSD) is to supply a range of sterile items to theatres, wards and other departments. Dressings and other soft packs may be made up of items or materials which are purchased sterile or unsterile or prepared in the department. The department will also clean and sterilize equipment for re-use, e.g. theatre instruments. HSSDs should operate whenever possible according to the guidelines produced by the DHSS for Good Manufacturing Practice (GMP)[68]. To minimize the risk of transfer of infection from 'sterilized' items rigorous attention must be paid to the control of the sterilization process. The frequency and methods of testing are described in detail in HTM10. Environmental control in other areas, e.g. for preparation of items prior to sterilization, can be excessive leading to unnecessarily frequent cleaning of surfaces and the provision of air filtered to unnecessarily low particle sizes and at higher than required flow rates. Such procedures can substantially increase costs and be limiting in the range of items supplied. There is no evidence of infection caused by inadequate environmental control when items have been subsequently sterilized effectively.

The HSSD may also include a Hospital Disinfection Unit (HDU). The function of this unit is to reprocess permanent medical equipment for re-use. This will usually involve cleaning, disinfection and checking that the equipment is functioning correctly. Medical equipment is becoming increasingly complex and requires specialized skills and equipment to reprocess. For economical reasons these facilities cannot be made available in each ward and department, and centralizing is often necessary. To ensure that equipment is functioning after cleaning and disinfection, it may be necessary to consult the Biomedical Engineering Department as specialized test equipment and additional skills may be required. It is, therefore, preferable that the two departments are in close proximity.

Hospital staff have become increasingly concerned with the risk of acquiring infection, especially HBV and HIV. Hepatitis B infection can occur when quite small amounts of contaminated blood are introduced by contact with broken skin. Current evidence suggests that larger amounts of contaminated blood need to be introduced, usually by injection, to transfer HIV. Risk can be reduced by wearing gloves when handling blood-stained items and taking particular care when handling used, sharp instruments. Known high risk equipment should be decontaminated at the earliest possible stage after being brought into the HSSD, preferably before handling. All instruments, etc., that require washing should preferably be heat disinfected at this stage. For high risk instruments it may be possible to arrange for their return to the HSSD in a suitable container that could be placed directly into the washing machine. This is preferable to using chemical disinfectants which may themselves be a toxic hazard, or autoclaving instruments prior to washing. Autoclaving adds an additional stage and is likely to coagulate protein making it difficult to remove at the wash stage. Heat disinfection at the wash stage may also be advantageous for some anaesthetic equipment since it should then be possible to pack it on removal from the washer without any further procedures.

However, if washer/disinfectors are to be used for either of these purposes an improvement in standards of control is required. Agreement on acceptable cycles and methods of commissioning and regularly checking of machines is necessary. The coolest part of the most difficult load would need to reach a temperature of 90°C or be raised to 80°C and held for 1 minute or to 70°C for 3 minutes. These correspond to standards accepted for laundering[58].

It is recommended by the DHSS that certificates are issued stating that equipment returned for servicing or repair is microbiologically safe. However, any item, unless sterilized and packed, will be contaminated with a variable number of unknown organisms, and the risk of infection for any specific individual is related to his/her immunological status, which will usually be unknown. It would be inadvisable to give such an assurance. A further problem arises as to which equipment should be included in the category requiring a certificate. Risk associated with the repair of toilets and drains would theoretically be at least as high as from portable medical equipment, but giving an assurance on the safety of these items would be even more impractical.

The risk of transferring infection when handling medical equipment can be minimized if sensible procedures are routinely followed.

High risk equipment can be identified by the following criteria:

1. Contact with patients suffering from infections caused by pathogenic organisms not commonly found in the environment, e.g. *Salmonella* and other intestinal pathogens, *Mycobacterium tuberculosis,* HIV, HBV or other diseases or equipment designated as high risk by the microbiologist.
2. Visible soiling with blood, body fluids or excreta, e.g. suction, other respiratory and human waste disposal equipment.
3. Blood analysis equipment, which is likely to be contaminated with blood from a large number of patients.

**Procedures for handling and servicing all equipment irrespective of risk**

Wear impervious gloves and a plastic apron.
Remove all attached tubing and if disposable discard as clinical waste.
If non-disposable, arrange for heat disinfection.
Empty any reservoirs into a sluice sink taking care to minimize aerosol production.
Hand wash-basins or food preparation sinks should not be used.
If the reservoir is removable, heat disinfect in a washer/disinfector.
If not removable, wipe and dry.
Wipe all outside surfaces and any internal surfaces likely to have been in contact with blood or secretions with a detergent solution using a disposable wipe, and dry.

**Procedures for high risk equipment**

It may be possible to decontaminate the entire item of equipment in a low temperature steam autoclave, an ethylene oxide chamber or a formalin cabinet. Small items of equipment can be immersed in 2% glutaraldehyde for 10 minutes, but this is a potentially toxic agent and suitable precautions must be taken (see p. 87). However, these processes should not be attempted unless it is certain the equipment will withstand the process. Outside surfaces can be decontaminated by wiping with alcohol or a 1% clear soluble phenolic solution. It is often not possible to disinfect all the potentially contaminated interior surfaces without damaging the equipment, invalidating any guarantee or service contract. Detailed written protocols should be developed in consultation with the microbiologist for each item of equipment as the need develops.

It is, however, not usually possible to guarantee that all internal surfaces have been decontaminated and a note should be attached to all high risk equipment as follows:

'This equipment has been cleaned and disinfected, but because of the complexity all internal surfaces may not have been treated. Although the risk from infection is low we would advise the following precautions when disassembling:

1. Wear impervious (rubber) gloves, and a plastic apron to protect the clothing.
2. If any tubing or reservoirs contain fluid, empty first, rinse and immerse for 10 minutes in a freshly prepared 1% solution of a clear soluble phenolic or 1% bleach* then rinse and dry.
3. Visibly soiled surfaces should be wiped with one of the above solutions or 70% alcohol.
4. Always wash your hands after completing a work session and before eating or smoking.'

For other items:
'This equipment has not been used on a patient with a known high risk infection, and it has been cleaned. To avoid the minimal risk involved in handling any equipment that has been in close contact with hospital patients, the same precautions are required as for equipment from high risk patients.'

# Intensive care units

Infections are mainly due to Gram-negative bacilli, e.g. *Klebsiella* spp., *Ps. aeruginosa, Serratia marcescens, Acinetobacter anitratum,* as well as *Staph. aureus.* The dry environment, e.g. walls, floors and ceilings, do not require any particular attention. A single-bedded ventilated cubicle suitable for source or protective isolation is advised if the unit has an open plan layout. Beds should be as far apart as possible (e.g. over 3 metres) so that large droplets from the respiratory tract of one patient do not reach the adjacent patients, as well as allowing sufficient room for equipment and attention by staff. A plenum ventilation system is not required to prevent the spread of infection but may be necessary to provide a suitable

*Do not use bleach on metal surfaces.

working environment; 8–12 air changes per hour should be sufficient. Wash-basins should be conveniently placed for staff attending any patient and should be well designed (see Chapter 8).

Medical equipment can be an important source of infection[44,46]. Ease of decontamination should be considered when buying new equipment. Methods of decontamination and frequency of cleaning should be defined and preferably carried out in an equipment cleaning and disinfection department. Static fluids or wet equipment, e.g. disinfectant solutions containing tubing, nailbrushes, mops, washing bowls should not be kept in the unit. Gowns and masks are not usually necessary, but may be worn when carrying out suction procedures, and a separate gown or apron should be used for attending an infectious patient. Overshoes and hats are unnecessary and sticky or disinfectant mats at the entrance to the unit are of no value (see p. 124).

Handwashing is the most important technique and requires particular attention if staff move from one patient to another. Although plain soap is adequate, an antiseptic detergent, e.g. povidone-iodine or chlorhexidine, may be preferred; 70% ethyl or 60% isopropyl alcohol with 1% glycerol is a rapid and effective method of hand disinfection and is particularly useful in an ITU. Gloves should be worn for suction and other contaminated procedures.

However, reasonable care will eliminate or considerably reduce exogenous infection and the problem of endogenous infections remains. These are mainly due to Gram-negative bacilli colonizing the mouth and gastrointestinal tract which may be aspirated into the lower respiratory tract[69]. A possible new approach is selective decontamination of the gastrointestinal tract by the use of topical polymyxin, tobramycin and amphotericin B and of systemic cefotaxime. Although preliminary reports look promising, the long-term potential hazards of superinfection and emergence of resistant strains remain[70]. Microbiological monitoring is necessary if such techniques are introduced and patients should be selected with care.

# Operating theatres[71–73]

The main factors associated with wound infection are considered in Chapter 5. The physical environment is of minor importance as a source of infection and frequent cleaning of walls and ceilings is unnecessary (2–4 times a year should be adequate). Routine disinfection of floors is not necessary for reasons already mentioned, but if a disinfectant is used, it should be rinsed off frequently; the dried deposit (also of detergents) may affect the antistatic properties of the floor. However, antistatic floors are unnecessary if explosive anaesthetic gases are never used.

A plenum ventilation system providing 20 air changes per hour should be satisfactory for routine surgery and high efficiency filters are not required. Although the filters should be as close as possible to the outlet of the ducts this is not always possible; disinfection of ducts with formaldehyde is not necessary. If the system is shut off overnight, the ventilation system should be run for at least 30 minutes before using the operating room to remove any free particles. Measuring the air flow at regular intervals is of greater value than bacteriological sampling. Smoke tests are also useful to determine air flows through doorways. The air should flow from the operating room outwards, apart from into the clean preparation room which should have the same or slightly higher air flow. It is important to remember that the operating room during an operation probably has more bacteria in the air than any other room in the suite, apart from changing rooms before and after operating lists.

Humidification systems should be of a steam injection type if possible, since Gram-negative bacilli will grow in most other systems, particularly if recirculation of water is involved. Nevertheless, the risk of airborne transfer of organisms from a humidifier to the theatre is small. Filters will further reduce this possibility.

Infection risks from bacteria on floors are small and there is little advantage in having a transfer area and changing trolleys, or putting on overshoes. The patient may be transferred directly from the ward to operating room in a bed, provided ward bedding is removed before entering the operating room. Adhesive or disinfectant mats should be avoided. Tests have shown that these mats do not significantly reduce the number of bacteria on the floor of the operating room[6]. If the mats are not regularly changed, anaerobic spore-bearing bacilli, e.g. *Clostridium welchii* may accumulate and could actually be transferred to shoes or trolleys.

Nevertheless, it is rational for all persons entering the clean area of the theatre to change completely into clean clothing and put on theatre shoes or boots. Although ordinary theatre clothing and cotton gowns allow bacteria to escape into the environment, most of the organisms (e.g. *Staph. epidermidis* and diphtheroids) are unlikely to cause infection except in implant surgery. Bacteria-impermeable clothing (ventilated if necessary) may be preferable for high risk surgery, possibly associated with a laminar flow system[23, 71]. Wearing of masks does not reduce the number of airborne organisms and probably has little effect on the infection rate, but again it is rational if masks are considered necessary for the operating team to wear efficient filter-type masks; wearing of make-up or wedding rings is probably a very minor infection risk. However, it is rational to prevent unnecessary people entering the theatre suite, particularly the operating room, and to maintain hygienic discipline without too much ritual. Disinfection of the surgeon's hand and the operation site is also rational and has a proven bacteriological effect[74, 75]. Routine environmental bacteriological monitoring is unnecessary, but air sampling in commissioning new theatres may be advisable for legal rather than microbiological reasons.

# Special care baby units[73]

The common organisms causing infection are *E.coli, Klebsiella* spp., *Ps. aeruginosa,* Lancefield group B streptococci, *Staph. aureus* and less frequently *Serratia marcescens* and *Acinetobacter anitratum*. Group B streptococci are generally acquired from the mother during delivery but cross-infection can occur in the nursery. Colonization of the mouth and intestinal tract with Gram-negative bacilli is common. Infection mainly spreads from baby to baby on the hands of staff. Masks are unnecessary and individual gowns are only needed for handling infected babies or during outbreaks. An antiseptic detergent preparation is usually advised for handwashing but, as in the ITU, disinfection with alcohol is particularly convenient when moving rapidly from one baby to another. Communal pots of ointments or creams should be avoided.

Incubators should be washed and dried after use by each baby; special attention should be paid to rubber seals, mattresses and the humidifier[76]. Gram-negative bacilli surviving or growing on moist surfaces are the main hazards in baby incubators, and drying after cleaning is the main method of control. Disinfection is not usually necessary, but wiping over or spraying with 70% alcohol after cleaning should be satisfactory if disinfection is required and it does not damage the incubator. Wiping over the cleaned incubator with a weak hypochlorite solution (125 ppm available chlorine) is also effective, but it should be rinsed off with water. Incubators can be conveniently cleaned in an equipment cleaning and disinfection section of the HSSD.

Other items requiring regular cleaning or disinfection are suction and respiratory equipment, aerosol humidifiers, rectal thermometers, and intragastric feeding equipment and baths. Infant feeds should, if possible, be sterile and expressed milk should be pasteurized and monitored bacteriologically. The pasteurizer should be regularly checked to ensure temperatures and times are correct. In addition to pasteurization of the milk, donors of expressed breast milk should be checked for HIV antibody.

## Protective isolation units

These are commonly available for immunosuppressed patients, e.g. with organ transplants or leukaemia. Infections are mainly endogenous and tend to be caused by *E.coli, Klebsiella* spp., *Bacteroides* spp., *Staph. aureus,* cytomegalovirus and *Candida. Ps. aeruginosa* is a problem in some units.

A single room (with or without a ventilation system) is usually adequate provided barrier nursing procedures and techniques are good and doors are kept closed. If ventilation is required a plenum system providing 8–12 changes per hour should be adequate. However, the value of single room protective isolation remains doubtful[77].

In the authors' own unit, masks, caps and overshoes are not worn and there has been little evidence of transfer of infection over a period of 10 years[38]. Gowns or plastic aprons are worn and kept within the room for 1 day before changing. In some units, particularly those concerned with cardiac and bone marrow transplants, precautions are often much stricter and involve full protective clothing or plastic isolators and possibly a laminar flow system. The advantages of these complex precautions remain uncertain. There is also some evidence that oral non-absorbable antibiotics (e.g. framycetin, colistin, nystatin) help to reduce the number of infections in high risk patients, e.g. with leucocytes lower than 1000/mm$^3$ but again there is some uncertainty. Routine bacteriological monitoring of patients is also controversial[78]. The unit should have suitable equipment for disinfecting cutlery and crockery and bedpans, preferably by heat. Uncooked foods, especially salads, may contain large numbers of *Pseudomonas, Klebsiella* or *Listeria* and should be avoided in high risk patients.

General hospitals can rarely afford to staff a special protective isolation unit, but source and protective isolation patients can be nursed in the same unit provided hygienic measures are efficient and the direction of the air flow in the cubicles can be changed as necessary[38, 79].

*Appendix 1*

# Notes on infections

| Disease | Incubation period | Period of infectivity | Action required for hospital contacts | Restriction of admissions | Category of isolation or precautions | Comments |
|---------|-------------------|----------------------|--------------------------------------|---------------------------|--------------------------------------|----------|
| *AIDS* (see Human immunodeficiency virus infection) | | | | | | |
| *Anthrax* Cutaneous | 1–7 days (usually 2) | Until lesions are free from anthrax bacilli. No evidence of person-to-person spread from cutaneous lesions | None | Consult Infection Control Officer | Wound/secretion | Inform factory inspectors where necessary. Inform veterinary authorities |
| Pulmonary | | | | | Respiratory | |
| *Bornholm disease* (pleurodynia) | 3–5 days | During acute stage | None | None | None | |
| *Brucellosis* | Variable, usually 7–21 days | Person to person transmission not known | None | None | Secretion, if draining lesion | |
| *Campylobacter diarrhoea* | 1–10 days | Not usually transmitted from person to person | None | None | Excretion | |
| *Candidiasis* | Variable | Duration of illness. Spread rare, except in neonates | None | None | Secretion (?) in neonates | |
| *Carditis* (viral) | 3–8 days | During acute stage | None | None | Depends on specific infectious agent | |
| *Chicken-pox* | 11–21 days (usually 13–17) | 7 days after onset of rash | Gammaglobulin for susceptible patients | Immune patients only admitted | Respiratory or home if suitable | |

| Disease | Incubation period | Period of infectivity | Action for contacts | Restrictions | Type of isolation | Notes |
|---|---|---|---|---|---|---|
| Cholera | Few hours to 5 days (usually 2–3 days) | Until stools are negative | None | No restrictions after isolation of infected patients | Enteric | Notify laboratory before swabbing contacts. (Close contact – within touching distance of case during period of infection) |
| Diphtheria | 2–7 days | From onset until culture of 3 consecutive nose and throat swabs are negative following acute stage | Nose and throat swabs from all contacts. Prophlyactic erythromycin may be given to close contacts | No admissions until contacts bacteriologically clear | Respiratory | |
| Dysentery Bacillary | 1–6 days | Until culture of stool negative | Search for missed cases and carriers if hospital-acquired | Usually no restrictions after isolation of infected patients | Enteric or home if suitable | Staff cases (except catering staff) return to work when free of symptoms but not to handle food or drugs until bacteriologically clear |
| Amoebic | 5 days to 3–4 weeks | As long as cysts appear in faeces | None | None | Excretion | Infection not initiated in temperate climate |
| Encephalitis (encephalomyelitis) | 4 days to several weeks according to causative virus | According to causative virus | None | None | Secretion(?) | |
| Enteric fever Typhoid Paratyphoid | 6–21 days | 6 consecutive negative stools | Search for contacts and carriers if hospital acquired | None | Enteric and blood | Cases occurring in hospitals – check for carriers, especially in catering staff |
| Food poisoning Staphylococcal Clostridial | 1–6 hours 6–12 hours | Not transmitted from person to person | None | None | | |
| Gas gangrene | 2–7 days or more | Not transmitted from person to person | None | None | Wound | Usually autogenous |

| Disease | Incubation period | Period of infectivity | Action required for hospital contacts | Restriction of admissions | Category of isolation or precautions | Comments |
|---|---|---|---|---|---|---|
| Glandular fever (infectious mononucleosis) | 11–15 days – may be longer | Uncertain until acute phase is over | None | None | Secretion (?) | Value of barrier nursing uncertain |
| Gram-negative bacilli (multi-resistant) | Variable | Until bacteriologically negative | None | None | Skin/wound or excretion (urine) | Single-room isolation for infection with highly resistant strains |
| Haemolytic streptococcal infections | 1–5 days | Until bacteriologically clear (or 24–48 h after starting therapy) | Search for source of infection in outbreak | No restriction – unless outbreak | Wound, skin secretion or respiratory – depending on site of infection | Transmission usually eliminated within 24 h of starting adequate penicillin therapy |
| Helminths Hookworm Roundworm Threadworm Tapeworm Whipworm | From few weeks to few months | As long as infestation lasts | None | None | Excretion | |
| Hepatitis HAV | 10–14 days | Commonly 7 days before to 7 days after onset | Close contacts may be given gamma-globulin | None | Excretion | Virus may persist in stools for months |
| HBV | 1–6 months | Virus may persist for years in blood | None | None | Single room and blood precautions for cases and carriers in renal and maternity units. Blood precautions for carriers in general wards | Special care in disposal of sharps. Hyperimmune gammaglobulin and vaccine |

| Disease | Incubation period | Infectious period | Prophylaxis/Immunization | Restrictions | Isolation/Secretion | Comments |
|---|---|---|---|---|---|---|
| Herpes simplex (including congenital herpes) | 4–5 days | Until vesicles healed | Gammaglobulin to children with eczema | None | Secretion | Protect immunologically compromised patients. Staff with cold sores not to work with compromised patients, neonates or burns patients |
| Herpes zoster | Unknown | Until healed | Protect compromised patients | Restrict to patients immune to chicken-pox | Respiratory and secretion | As herpes simplex, may lead to cases of chicken-pox |
| Human immunodeficiency virus (HIV) | Variable; acute viral infection 1–2 weeks, AIDS 2–15 years (median 8) | Virus persists in blood indefinitely | None | None | Blood | Contact Infection Control Officer |
| Impetigo | 1–3 days | Until bacteriologically clear | None (apart from surveillance) | None | Wound and skin | |
| Influenza | 1–4 days (usually 2) | In prodromal phase and for 3 days after onset | Immunization available | Restrict admissions unless unavoidable | Isolation precautions – doubtful value in epidemic | Staff with influenza should report sick |
| Lassa fever and related exotic fevers | 3–21 days | While symptoms persist | Consult Infection Control Officer | Consult Infection Control Officer | Strict | Notify Infection Control Officer immediately |
| Legionnaires' disease | 2–10 days (usually 5–6) | Not transmitted from person to person | None | None | Secretion | Contact Infection Control Officer re environmental investigation |
| Leptospirosis (Weil's disease) | 4–14 days (usually 10) | Not usually transmitted person to person | None | None | Excretion (urine only) | |
| Malaria | Variable | Not directly transmitted person to person | None | None | None | Care when handling sharps |

| Disease | Incubation period | Period of infectivity | Action required for hospital contacts | Restriction of admissions | Category of isolation or precautions | Comments |
|---|---|---|---|---|---|---|
| Measles | 6–12 days (usually 10) | 7 days from onset of rash | Human gammaglobulin for prophylaxis | Restrict to immune patients | Respiratory | Discharge home when possible |
| Meningitis (viral) | 3–10 days (for enterovirus infections) | Until virus no longer present in stools | None | None | Respiratory and excretion | |
| Meningococcal meningitis | 2–10 days (usually 3–4) | 24–28 hours after starting treatment | Usually none. Contact Infection Control Officer | None unless hospital outbreak | Respiratory | Home: close contacts treat with rifampicin |
| Mumps | 12–28 days (usually 18) | 7 days before to 9 days after onset of paratoid swelling | Non-immune male staff should avoid contact | No restriction for children. No admission for susceptible adults | Respiratory | Persons with subclinical infection may be infectious. Inform parents of new admissions to children's wards |
| Ophthalmia neonatorum (gonococcal) | 3–9 days | Until gonococcus eradicated – usually 24 hours from start of specific chemotherapy | Mother usually source. Treat and advise visit to VD clinic for contact tracing | None | Secretion. Single room with mother | |
| Poliomyelitis | 3–35 days (usually 10–15) | Until virus no longer present in stools | Gammaglobulin for non-immune contacts. Booster for immunized contacts | Immunized patients only | Respiratory and enteric | No elective surgery on non-immunized contacts. Avoid i.m. injections if possible |
| Puerperal sepsis (see Haemolytic streptococcal disease) | | | | Wound, single room | | |
| Rubella Adult | 14–21 days | 7 days from onset of rash | Female: test blood for antibodies within 5 days. Notify obstretrician of any pregnant, non-immune women | No admission during first 4 months of pregnancy | Respiratory or home if suitable | Inform other patients and all staff. Warn non-immune women of child-bearing age |

| | | | | | | |
|---|---|---|---|---|---|---|
| Newborn | | 6 months or longer | As above | | Respiratory and excretion | |
| *Salmonella* | 12 hours to 3 days | Until culture of stool negative (less after acute stage) | Usually none. Contact Infection Control Officer | None unless outbreak in hospital | Enteric | Staff (except catering) return to work when free of symptoms but not to handle drugs or food until bacteriologically clear |
| *Staphylococcal infections (not multi-resistant)* | | | | | | |
| Pneumonia | Variable | Until bacteriologically negative | None | None | Respiratory | |
| Skin/wound | | While lesions persist | None | None | Skin/wound | Single room if patient is heavy dispenser |
| *Multi-resistant strains* (especially resistant to methicillin, fusidic acid and gentamicin) | Variable | Until bacteriologically negative | Variable. Consult Infection Control Officer | None unless outbreak | Skin/wound | High priority for a single room, especially MRSA in high risk units |
| *Tetanus* | Variable (usually 7–10 days) | Not infective | None | None | None | |
| *Tuberculosis* (open respiratory) | Variable (about 4–6 weeks) | Usually about 2 weeks after start of treatment | Monitor close contacts | None | Respiratory | |
| *Whooping cough* | 21 days (usually less than 10) | 7 days before to 3 weeks from onset of cough | Discharge non-immune when possible | Restrict to immune patients | Respiratory or home if suitable | Prophylactic erythromycin to close contacts under 1 year |

## Explanation of categories of precautions

### Wound and skin precautions

To prevent transfer of organisms from infected wounds or skin, and from items in immediate contact with the infected site:

1. Handwashing immediately before and after all contact with the infected patient, and any item likely to have come into contact with the infected site, e.g. bedding, used dressings, etc.
2. Dressings: use aseptic technique and wear gloves. Disposable plastic apron required for direct patient contact only. Seal discarded dressing in plastic bag immediately after removal.
3. Bed linen: avoid unnecessary agitation when removing. Seal in impervious bag on removal and remove from patient environment promptly.

No other special precautions required.

These precautions are mainly required for purulent wound infections or skin infections such as impetigo and for exfoliative skin conditions with a concurrent infection and where the infective agent is *Staph. aureus*, particularly if the strain is resistant to several antibiotics. Also may be required for streptococcal and highly resistant Gram-negative infections.

### Excretion and secretion precautions

To prevent the transfer of potentially pathogenic microbes from the excretions or secretions produced by infected patients and may include blood, pus, urine, faeces and sputum.

1. Wear gloves when handling.
2. Seal contaminated material in impervious bag or other suitable container as soon as possible.
3. Dispose of promptly; do not store without adequate security. Final disposal should kill microbes, e.g. burning, or provide sufficient dilution to render safe, e.g. disposal directly into sewage.
4. Any item in contact with the excretions and secretions that is to be re-used should be adequately disinfected, preferably by heat, before re-use, e.g. bedpans, urinals, bed linen.

### Enteric

As excretion, single room if possible.

### Respiratory

As secretion, single room (see also Chapter 6).

# References

1. Meers, P. D., Ayliffe, G. A. J., Emmerson, A. M. *et al.* (1981) Report of the National Survey of Infection in hospitals – 1980. *J. Hosp. Infect.* (supplement)
2. Ayliffe, G. A. J. (1971) In: *Proceedings of the International Conference on Nosocomial Infections, 1970, Chicago,* American Hospital Association, pp. 282–284
3. DHSS (1988) *Hospital Infection Control – Guidance on the Control of Infection in Hospitals.* Prepared by the DHSS/PHLS Hospital Infection Working Group.
4. Haley, R. W., Culver, D. H., White, J. W. *et al.* (1985) The efficacy of infection surveillance and control programs in preventing nosocomial infection in US hospital. *Am. J. Epidemiol.* **121**: 182
5. Pettit, F. and Lowbury, E. J. L. (1968) Survival of wound pathogens under different environmental conditions. *J. Hyg. (Lond.)* **66**: 393
6. Ayliffe, G. A. J., Collins, B. J. and Lowbury, E. J. L. (1967) Ward floors and other surfaces as reservoirs of hospital infection. *J. Hyg. (Lond.)* **65**: 515
7. Clark, S., Lach, V. and Lidwell, O. M. (1981) The performance of the Biotest RCS centrifugal air sampler. *J. Hosp. Infect.* **2**: 181
8. Lowbury, E. J. L., Thom, B. T., Lilly, H. A. *et al.* (1970) Sources of infection with *Pseudomonas aeruginosa* in patients with tracheostomy. *J. Med. Microbiol.* **3**: 39
9. Blair, J. E. and Williams, R. E. O. (1961) Phage typing of staphylococci. *Bull. WHO* **24**: 771
10. Govan, J. R. W. (1978) In: Bergan, T. and Norris, J. R. (eds) *Methods in Microbiology – 10,* London, New York, San Francisco, Academic Press, p. 61
11. Elek, S. D. and Conen, P. E. (1975) The virulence of *Staphylococcus pyogenes* for man. A study of the problems of wound infection. *Br. J. Exp. Pathol.* **38**: 573
12. Ayliffe, G. A. J., Babb, J. R. and Collins, B. J. (1973) In: Hers, P. H. and Winkler, K. C. (eds) *Airborne Transmission and Airborne Infection,* Utrecht, Dosthoek Publishing Company, p. 435
13. Blowers, R., Hill, J. and Howell, A. (1973) In: Hers, P. H. and Winkler, K. C. (eds) *Airborne Transmission and Airborne Infection,* Utrecht, Dosthoek Publishing Company, p. 432
14. Ayliffe, G. A. J. (1988) Hospital infection surveillance in the United Kingdom. *Infect. Control Hosp. Epidemiol.* **9**: 320
15. Ayliffe, G. A. J. (1978) In: Bergan, T. and Norris, J. R. (eds) *Methods in Microbiology – 10,* London, New York, San Francisco, Academic Press, p. 39
16. Report of a combined working party of the Hospital Infection Society and the British Society of Antimicrobial Chemotherapy (1986) Guidelines for the control of epidemic methicillin resistant *Staphylococcus aureus. J. Hosp. Infect.* **7**: 193
17. Department of Health and Social Security Committee of Enquiry (1986) *First Report of the Committee of Inquiry into the Outbreak of Legionnaires' Disease in Stafford in April 1985,* London, HMSO
18. Advisory Committee on Dangerous Pathogens (1986) *LAV/HTLV III – The Causative Agents of AIDS and Related Conditions, Revised Guidelines,* London, HMSO
19. DHSS (1986) *Memorandum on the Control of Viral Haemorrhagic Fevers,* London, HMSO
20. Ayliffe, G. A. J., Brightwell, K. M., Collins, B. J. *et al.* (1977) Surveys of hospital infection in the Birmingham region. *J. Hyg. (Lond.)* **79**: 299
21. Cruse, P. J. E. and Foord, R. (1973) A five year prospective study of 23 649 surgical wounds. *Arch. Surg.* **107**: 206
22. Bibby, B. A., Collins, B. J. and Ayliffe, G. A. J. (1986) A mathematical model for assessing the risk of postoperative wound infection. *J. Hosp. Infect.* **8**: 31

23. Lidwell, O. M., Lowbury, E. J. L., Whyte, W. *et al.* (1983) The effect of ultraclean air in operating rooms on deep sepsis in the joint after total hip or knee replacement: a randomised study. *Br. Med. J.* **285**, 10

24. Ayliffe, G. A. J., Noy, M. E., Davies, J. G. *et al.* (1983) A comparison of pre-operative bathing with chlorhexidine-detergent and non-medicated soap in the prevention of wound infection. *J. Hosp. Infect.* **4**: 237

25. Hayek, L. J., Emmerson, J. M. and Gardner, A. M. N. (1987) A placebo-controlled trial on the effect of two pre-operative baths or showers with chlorhexidine-detergent on postoperative wound infection rates. *J. Hosp. Infect.* **10**: 165

26. Rotter, M. L., Larsen, S. O., Cooke, E. M. *et al.* (1988) A comparison of the effects of pre-operative whole-body bathing with detergent alone and with detergent containing chlorhexidine-gluconate in the frequency of wound infections after clean surgery. The European Working Party on Control of Hospital Infections. *J. Hosp. Infect.* **11**: 310

27. Seropian, R. and Reynolds, M. (1971) Wound infections after pre-operative depilatory versus razor preparations. *Am. J. Surg.* **121**: 251

28. Craven, D. E., Connolly, M. G., Lightenberg, D. A. *et al.* (1982) Contamination of mechanical ventilators with tubing changes every 24 and 48 hours. *N. Engl. J. Med.* **306**: 1505

29. Slade, N. and Gillespie, W. A. (1985) *The Urinary Tract and the Catheter: Infection and other Problems,* Chichester, New York, Wiley

30. Gillespie, W. A. (1963) In: Williams, R. E. O. and Shooter, R. A. (eds) *Infection in Hospitals, Epidemiology and Control,* Oxford, Blackwell, p. 109

31. Ayliffe, G. A. J., Babb, J. R., Davies, J. G. and Lilly, H. A. (1988) Hand disinfection: a comparison of various agents in laboratory and ward studies. *J. Hosp. Infect.* **11**: 226

32. Taylor, L. J. (1978) An evaluation of handwashing techniques (Parts 1 and 2). *Nursing Times,* January 12th and 19th, pp. 54, 108

33. Ayliffe, G. A. J., Babb, J. R. and Quoraishi, A. H. (1978) A test for hygienic hand disinfection. *J. Clin. Path.* **31**: 923

34. Thomlinson, D. (1987) To clean or not to clean. *J. Infect. Control Nurs.* **35**: 71

35. Maki, D. G. and Ringer, M. (1987) Evaluation of dressing regimens for the prevention of infection with peripheral intravenous catheters. *JAMA* **258**: 239

36. Simpson, R. A. (1986) Systemic and topical antimicrobial agents in the prevention of catheter associated bacteriuria and its consequences. *Infect. Control* (suppl.) **7**: 100

37. Bagshawe, K. D., Blowers, R. and Lidwell, O. M. (1978) Isolating patients in hospital to control infection. *Br. Med. J.* **2**: 609, 634, 744, 808, 879

38. Ayliffe, G. A. J., Babb, J. R., Taylor, L. *et al.* (1979) A unit for source and protective isolation in a general hospital. *Br. Med. J.* **2**: 461

39. Haley, R. W., Garner, J. S. and Simmons, B. P. (1985) A new approach to the isolation of hospitalized patients with infectious diseases: alternative systems. *J. Hosp. Infect.* **6**: 128

40. Gallagher, J., Strangeways, J. E. M., Allt-Graham, J. (1987) Contamination control in long-term ventilation. *Anaesthesia* **42**: 476

41. Ayliffe, G. A. J., Babb, J. R. and Collins, B. J. (1974) Carpets in hospital wards. *Br. Hosp. J. Soc. Serv. Rev.* October

42. Ayliffe, G. A. J., Collins, B. J. and Lowbury, E. J. L. (1966) Cleaning and disinfection of hospital floors. *Br. Med. J.* **2**: 442

43. Ayliffe, G. A. J., Babb, J. R., Collins, B. J. *et al.* (1974) *Pseudomonas* in hospital sinks. *Lancet,* **2**: 578

44. Hovig, B. (1981) Lower respiratory tract infections associated with respiratory therapy and anaesthesia equipment. *J. Hosp. Infect.* **2**: 301

45. Holdcroft, A., Lumley, J., Gaya, H. *et al.* (1974) Respiratory filters in clinical practice. *Lancet,* **2**: 25

46. Phillips, I. and Spencer, G. (1965) *Pseudomonas aeruginosa* cross-infection due to contaminated respiratory apparatus. *Lancet* **2**: 1325

47. Deverill, C. E. A. and Dutt, K. K. (1980) Methods of decontamination of anaesthetic equipment: daily sessional exchange of circuits. *J. Hosp. Infect.* **1**: 165

48. O'Connor, H. J. and Axon, A. T. R. (1983) Gastrointestinal endoscopy: infection and disinfection. *Gut* **24**: 1067

49. Ayliffe, G. A. J., Babb, J. R. and Bradley, C. R. (1986) Disinfection of endoscopes. *J. Hosp. Infect.* **7**: 296

50. Babb, J. R. and Bradley, C. R. (1988) Decontamination of fibreoptic endoscopes: an update. *J. Sterile Services Management* April: 9

51. Tyler, R. and Ayliffe, G. A. J. (1987) A surface test for virucidal activity of disinfectants: preliminary study with herpes virus. *J. Hosp. Infect.* **9**: 22
52. Kelsey, J. C. (1972) The myth of surgical sterility. *Lancet.* **2**: 1301
53. Hurrell, D. J. (1987) Low-temperature steam and formaldehyde (LTSF) sterilization. Its effectiveness and merits. *J. Sterile Services Management.* **5**: 40
54. Alder, V. G. (1987) The formaldehyde/low temperature steam sterilizing procedure. *J. Hosp. Infect.* **9**: 194
55. Babb, J. R., Phelps, M., Downes, J. *et al.* (1982) Evaluation of an ethylene oxide sterilizer. *J. Hosp. Infect.* **3**: 385
56. Central Sterilizing Club, Working Party Report No. 2 (1986) Sterilization and disinfection of heat labile equipment. Obtainable from Hospital Infection Research Laboratory
57. Babb, J. R., Bradley, C. R. and Ayliffe, G. A. J. (1980) Sporicidal activity of glutaraldehydes and hypochlorites and other factors influencing their selection for the treatment of medical equipment. *J. Hosp. Infect.* **1**: 63
58. Central Sterilizing Club, Working Party Report No. 1 (1986) Washer/disinfection machines. Obtainable from Hospital Infection Research Laboratory
59. Ayliffe, G. A. J., Coates, D. and Hoffman, P. N. (1984) *Chemical Disinfection in Hospitals,* Public Health Laboratory Service, London
60. Coates, D. (1988) Comparison of sodium hypochlorite and sodium dichloroisocyanurate disinfectants. Neutralization by serum. *J. Hosp. Infect.* **11**: 60
61. Collins, B. J., Wilkins, M. and Ayliffe, G. A. J. (1972) Dry cleaning of hospital floors. *Br. Hosp. J. Soc. Serv. Rev.* December
62. Collins, B. J., Cripps, N. and Spooner, A. (1987) Controlling microbial decontamination levels. *Laundry and Cleaning News,* 30–31
63. Advisory Committee on Dangerous Pathogens (1984) *Categorization of Pathogens According to Hazard and Categories of Containment,* London, HMSO
64. DHSS (1987) *Health Service Catering Hygiene,* London, HMSO
65. *Report of the Committee of Enquiry into an Outbreak of Food Poisoning at Stanley Royd Hospital 1986,* London, HMSO
66. Sandys, G. H. and Wilkinson, P. J. (1988) Microbiological evaluation of a hospital delivered meals service using pre-cooked chilled foods. *J. Hosp. Infect.* **9**, 209
67. DHSS (1989) *Health Service Guidelines on Pre-cooked Chilled Foods,* London, HMSO
68. DHSS (1981) *Guide to Good Manufacturing Practices for Sterile Medical Devices and Surgical Products,* London, HMSO
69. Sanderson, P. J. (1986) The source of pneumonia in ITU patients. *Infect. Control* (suppl.) **7**: 10
70. Ledingham, I., Alcock, S., Eastaway, A. *et al.* (1988) Triple regime for selective decontamination of the digestive tract; systemic cefotaxime and microbiological surveillance for prevention of acquired infection in intensive care. *Lancet* **1**: 785
71. Sanderson, P. J. (ed.) (1988) Infection control in orthopaedic surgery: Symposium. *J. Hosp. Infect.* (suppl. C)
72. Ayliffe, G. A. J. and Lowbury, E. J. L. (1982) Airborne infection in hospital. *J. Hosp. Infect.* **3**: 217
73. Lowbury, E. J. L., Ayliffe, G. A. J., Geddes, A. M. *et al.* (1981) *Control of Hospital Infection. A Practical Handbook* 2nd edn, London, Chapman and Hall
74. Lowbury, E. J. L. (1982) In: Russell, A. D., Hugo, W. B. and Ayliffe, G. A. J. (eds) *Principles and Practice of Disinfection, Preservation and Sterilization,* Oxford, Blackwell Scientific Publications, p. 262
75. Ayliffe, G. A. J. (1984) Surgical scrub and skin disinfection. *Infect. Control* **5**: 23
76. Ayliffe, G. A. J., Collins, B. J. and Green, S. (1975) Hygiene of babies' incubators (correspondence). *Lancet.* **1**: 923
77. Nausef, W. M. and Maki, D. G. (1981) A study of simple protective isolation in patients with granulocytopenia. *N. Engl. J. Med.* **304**: 448
78. Daw, M. A., McMahon, E. and Keane, C. T. (1988) Surveillance cultures in the neutropenic patient. *J. Hosp. Infect.* **12**: 251
79. Rahman, M. (1985) Commissioning a new hospital isolation unit and assessment of its use over five years. *J. Hosp. Infect.* **6**: 65

# Bibliography

Altemeier, W. A., Burke, J. F., Privitt, B. A. *et al.* (ed. committee) (1984) *Manual on Control of Infection in Surgical Patients,* Philadelphia, Lippincott

Bartlett, C. L. R., Macrae, A. D. and Macfarlane, J. D. (1986) *Legionella Infections,* London, Arnold

Benenson, A. S. (ed.) (1985) *Control of Communicable Disease in Man,* 14th edn, New York, American Public Health Association

Bennett, J. V. and Brachman, P. S. (1986) *Hospital Infections,* 2nd edn, Boston, Little Brown

Castle, M. and Ajemiam, E. (1987) *Hospital Infection Control: Principles and Practice,* 2nd edn, Chichester, New York, Wiley

Christie, A. B. (1987) *Infectious Diseases. Epidemiology and Clinical Practice,* 4th edn, Edinburgh, Churchill Livingstone

Collee, J. P., Duguiol, J. P., Fraser, A. G. and Marmion, P. P. (eds) (1989) *Mackie and MacCartney's Practical Medical Microbiology,* 13th edn, Edinburgh, Churchill Livingstone

Gardner, J. F. and Peel, M. M. (1986) *Introduction to Sterilization and Disinfection,* Edinburgh, Churchill Livingstone

Haley, R. H. (ed.) (1986) *Managing Hospital Infection Control for Cost-Effectiveness,* Chicago, American Hospital Publishing

Hobbs, B. C. and Roberts, D. (1987) *Food Poisoning and Food Hygiene,* 5th edn, London, Arnold

Johnston, I. D. A. and Hunter, A. R. (eds) (1984) *The Design and Utilization of Operating Theatres,* London, Arnold

Lowbury, E. J. L., Ayliffe, G. A. J., Geddes, A. M. *et al.* (1981) *Control of Hospital Infection: A Practical Handbook,* 2nd edn, London, Chapman and Hall

Maurer, I. M. (1985) *Hospital Hygiene,* 3rd edn, London, Arnold

Parker, M. and Stucke, V. A. (1978) *Microbiology for Nurses,* London, Baillière Tindall

Russell, A. D., Hugo, W. B. and Ayliffe, G. A. J. (eds) *Principles and Practice of Disinfection, Preservation and Sterilization,* Oxford, Blackwell Scientific Publications

Shanson, D. C. (1989) *Microbiology in Clinical Practice,* 2nd edn, Bristol, Wright PSG

Slade, N. and Gillespie, W. A. (1985) *The Urinary Tract and the Catheter: Infection and Other Problems,* Chichester, New York, Wiley

Wenzel, R. P. (ed.) (1987) *Prevention and Control of Nosocomial Infections,* Baltimore, Wilkins and Wilkins

Williams, R. E. O., Blowers, R., Garrod, L. P. and Shooter, R. A. (eds) (1966) *Hospital Infection: Causes and Prevention,* 2nd edn, London, Lloyd-Luke

# Index